EXCUSE ME
Can I Eat That?

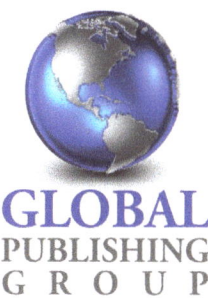

Global Publishing Group
Australia • New Zealand • Singapore • America • London

EXCUSE ME Can I Eat That?

Delicious plant-based recipes for those following a gluten free diet and those suffering IBS.

JODIE MARTIN

BHSc Nutritional Medicine

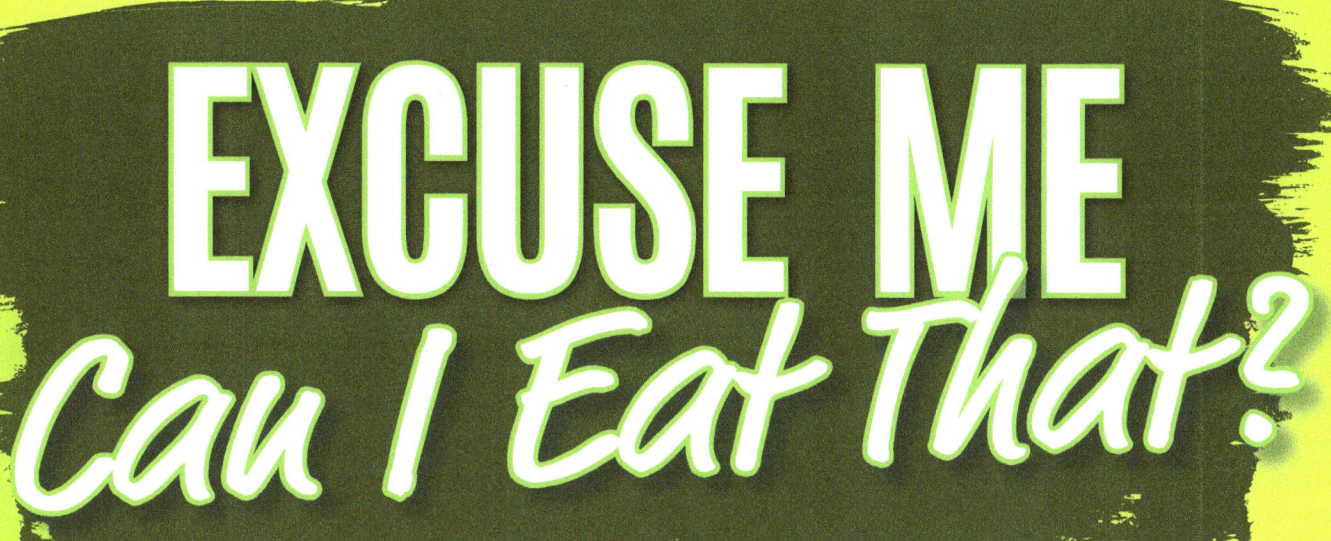

DISCLAIMER

All the information, techniques, skills and concepts contained within this publication are of the nature of general comment only and are not in any way recommended as individual advice. The intent is to offer a variety of information to provide a wider range of choices now and in the future, recognising that we all have widely diverse circumstances and viewpoints. Should any reader choose to make use of the information contained herein, this is their decision, and the contributors (and their companies), authors and publishers do not assume any responsibilities whatsoever under any condition or circumstances. It is recommended that the reader obtain their own independent advice.

First Edition 2022

Copyright © 2022 Jodie Martin

All rights are reserved. The material contained within this book is protected by copyright law, no part may be copied, reproduced, presented, stored, communicated or transmitted in any form by any means without prior written permission.

National Library of Australia
Cataloguing-in-Publication entry:

Excuse Me, Can I Eat That? - Jodie Martin

1st ed.
ISBN: 978-1-925370-04-1 (pbk.)

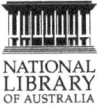 A catalogue record for this book is available from the National Library of Australia

Published by Global Publishing Group
PO Box 517 Mt Evelyn, Victoria 3796 Australia
Email Info@GlobalPublishingGroup.com.au

For further information about orders:
Phone: +61 3 9726 4133

I'd like to make special thanks to my husband David for his time, patience and dedication with getting this book together. I definitely could not have pulled this together without you.

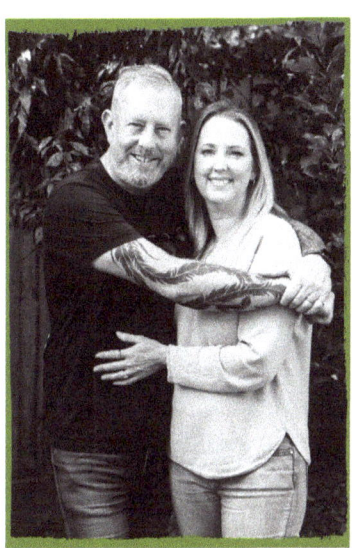

To my two wonderful children and partners, who did lots of taste testing for me, often the same dish over and over again until I felt I had it just right. Your patience has been overwhelming and I love you to bits.

To all my taste testers, this book would not be the same without you.

Jodie Martin

Be kind in thought, action, footprint and speech

Jodie Martin

TABLE OF CONTENTS

Conversion Tables	1
Introduction	2
My Journey to a Plant-based Diet	3
Fructose Malabsorption	5
Irritable Bowel Syndrome	6
Coeliac Disease	7
The Planter's Pantry	8

CHAPTER 1 BREAKFAST

Scrambled Tofu	12
Big Breakfast	15
Banana Pancakes	16
Coconut Flour Pancakes	19
Breakfast Smoothie	20
Green Smoothie	20
Breakfast on the Go	23
Breakfast Burrito	24
Creamy Quinoa Porridge	27

CHAPTER 2 SOUPS

Baked Pumpkin and Nutmeg Soup	30
Roasted Tomato and Basil Soup	33
Root Vegetable Soup	34
Miso Easy Soup	37
Minestrone	38
Oyster Mushroom Broth	41
Vietnamese Pho	42
Creamy Lentil Soup	45
Coconut and Sweet Potato Soup	46
Spinach Soup	49

CHAPTER 3 SALADS

Warm Summer Hemp Pasta Salad	52
Jewel Quinoa Salad	55
Smoked Paprika Roasted Pumpkin Salad	56
Old School Tropical Salad	58
Baba Ganoush	59
No-Egg Salad	60
Chickpea Tuna Salad	63
Peanut Soba Noodle Salad	64
Turmeric Rice	67
Zucchini and Hazelnut Salad with Walnut Vinaigrette	68

CHAPTER 4 STARTERS

Spinach Empanadas	72
Rosemary Polenta Chips	75
Nut Feta Stuffed Zucchini Flowers	76
Sundried Tomato and Feta Arancini Balls	79
Cucumber Bites	80
Bruschetta	83
Olive Tapenade	84
Sticky Tempeh Lettuce Boats	87
Satay Tofu Skewers	88
Carrot Sushi	91

CHAPTER 5 MAINS

Walnut Bolognaise	94
Easy-Peasy Tofu Steaks	97
Mexican Tofu Sticks	98
BBQ Pulled Jackfruit Sloppy Joe	101
Pumpkin Risotto	102
Spinach and Almond Roast	105
Tofu Spiced Couscous	106
Vegetable Curry with Coconut Rice	109
Retro Bubble and Squeak Patties	110
Cheesy Vegetable Bake	113

CHAPTER 6 DESSERTS

Baked Lemon Cheesecake with Raspberry Coulis	116
Chocolate Torte	119
Vanilla Slice	120
Chocolate Chip Cookies	123
Miso Salted Caramel	124
Banana Chocolate Bread	127
Butterscotch Pudding	128

CHAPTER 7 BITS AND PIECES

Macadamia Nut Pesto	133
Macadamia Feta	134
Salad Dressing	137
Tzatziki	138
Lime Salsa	141
'Not' Cheese Sauce	142
Walnut Vinaigrette	145
Sour Cream	146
Lemon Curd	149
Meet The Author	150
Recommended Resources	152

FREE BONUS GIFTS

Valued at $497 – But Yours **FREE!**

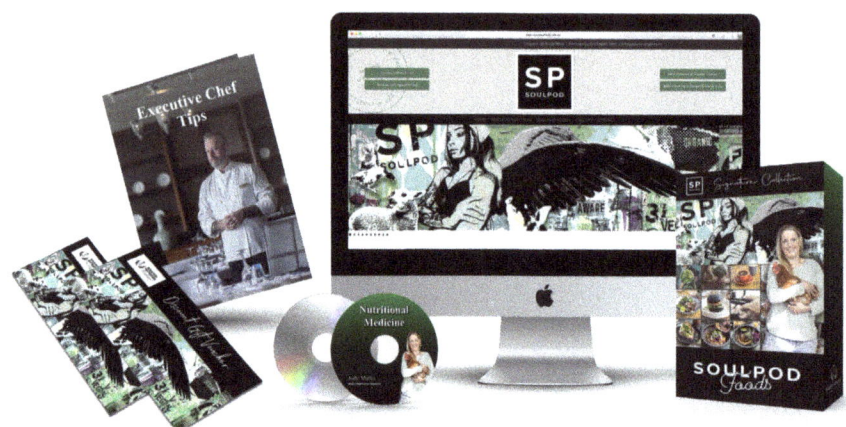

Claim your FREE BONUS GIFTS by going to
www.SoulpodFoods.com.au/Free-Gifts

Instant Access and FREE Download

We can't give you everything you need to know about Delicious plant-based foods in one small book.

So, we've created a very special website with loads of extra goodies, just for you. You'll find healthy recipes, diet plans, videos, checklists and meal vouchers.

So Enjoy! *Jodie xo*

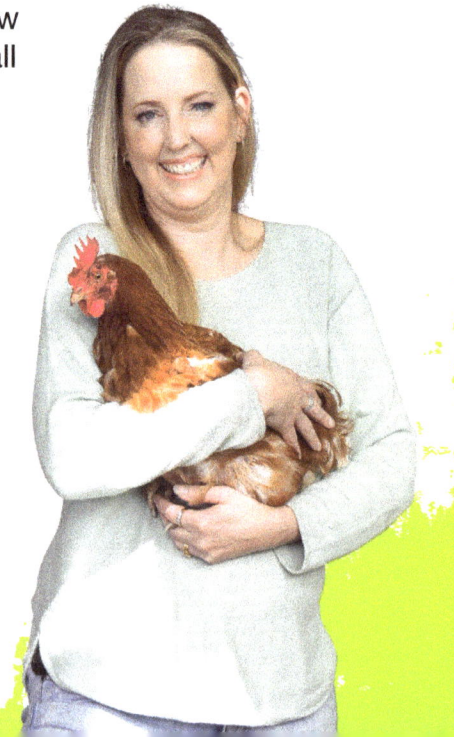

Claim your FREE BONUS GIFTS by going to
www.SoulpodFoods.com.au/Free-Gifts

CONVERSION TABLES

MEASUREMENT

CUP	ONCES	MILLILITERS	TBSP
8 cup	64 oz	1895 ml	128
6 cup	48 oz	1420 ml	96
5 cup	40 oz	1180 ml	80
4 cup	32 oz	960 ml	64
2 cup	16 oz	500 ml	32
1 cup	8 oz	250 ml	16
3/4 cup	6 oz	177 ml	12
2/3 cup	5 oz	158 ml	11
1/2 cup	4 oz	118 ml	8
3/8 cup	3 oz	90 ml	6
1/3 cup	2.5 oz	79 ml	5.5
1/4 cup	2 oz	59 ml	4
1/8 cup	1 oz	30 ml	3
1/16 cup	1/2 oz	15 ml	1

WEIGHT

IMPERIAL	METRIC
1/2 oz	15 g
1 oz	29 g
2 oz	57 g
3 oz	85 g
4 oz	113 g
5 oz	141 g
6 oz	170 g
8 oz	227 g
10 oz	283 g
12 oz	340 g
13 oz	369 g
14 oz	397 g
15 oz	425 g
1 lb	453 g

TEMPERATURE

FAHRENHEIT	CELSIUS
100 °F	37 °C
150 °F	65 °C
200 °F	93 °C
250 °F	121 °C
300 °F	150 °C
325 °F	160 °C
350 °F	180 °C
375 °F	190 °C
400 °F	200 °C
425 °F	220 °C
450 °F	230 °C
500 °F	260 °C
525 °F	274 °C
550 °F	288 °C

INTRODUCTION

I don't remember a time when I didn't have problems with my gut. My mum dragging me to doctor after doctor, with the same diagnosis – irritable bowel syndrome (IBS) and even, at one point, I was called a hypochondriac. As I got older, and the symptoms got worse – along with the psychological aspect of it all – it became very debilitating…

I wrote this book for all people out there with a similar story to mine.

It was after I became housebound, unable to work, that my husband reached panic point. After years of being told nothing was wrong with me, it was time to go see a gut specialist. With my husband by my side, off we went.

After the appropriate tests, we discovered I had coeliac disease – it was a relief to discover this, as it meant a change in diet would liberate me. My happiness was cut short when I continued to be not quite right. There were still the desperate dashes to the loo, the bloating, the pain, the fear of embarrassing myself in front of people with the noisier and smellier of symptoms, and an extremely foggy head. For four years after the coeliac diagnosis this continued.

A naturopath friend suggested I go and have a fructose and lactose breath test – which I did. The result came back that I was intolerant to both.

The fun begins… what do I eat now?!!

With the elimination of foods containing fructose and lactose I made quite a marked recovery and was able to enjoy life as I had before my illness.

When going out to eat, the question I most commonly asked was "What are the ingredients in that?" or, after explaining my conditions to confused wait staff, I'd ask what would be safe for me to eat… hence the title of this book!

It's a combination of all that which prompted me to progress with this book. I can't be the only coeliac, low FODMAP (fermentable oligosaccharides, disaccharides, monosaccharides and polyols!), IBS casualty vegan out there! Can I? As a nutritionist who loves to cook and has a chef husband, I felt it my privilege to put this book together. I have included some of our favourite yummy dishes that are full of flavour so you don't feel like you are missing out.

Bon Appetit

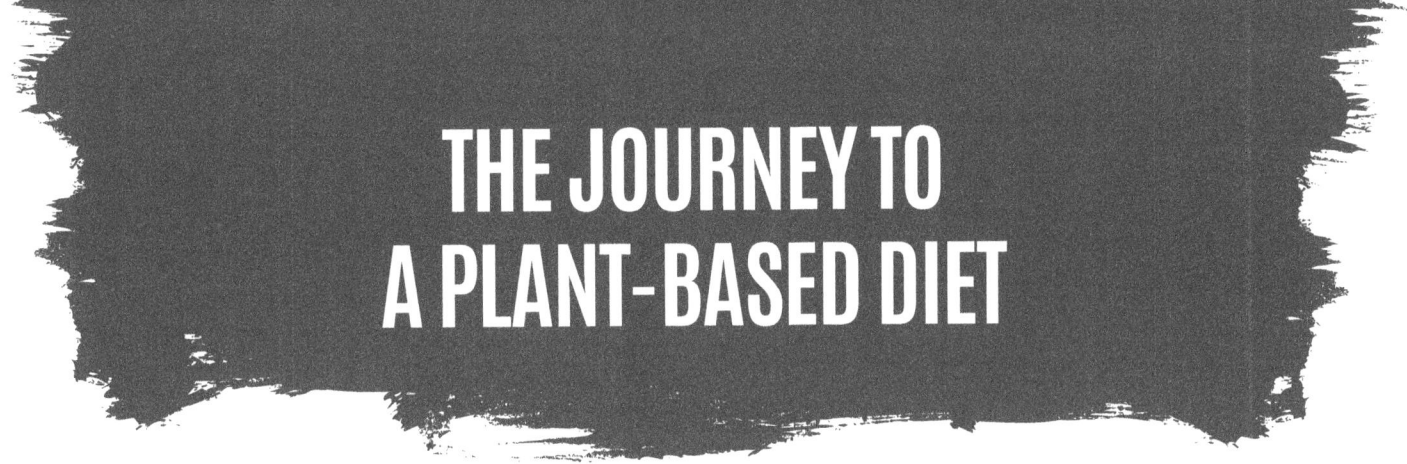

THE JOURNEY TO A PLANT-BASED DIET

As I sit here to write this book, I realise that a dream is close to coming true. To share with people my story and journey to veganism and share with you the delicious dishes that have become a daily eat in our house.

As a young girl, I never really took to eating meat. It never felt natural but, at the same time, I never gave much thought to how that animal got to my plate.

I adore animals, always have, but like so many people I would proudly say I loved them as I was digging into yoghurt, a piece of chicken or a cheese sandwich. One of my earliest memories was going on a church camp to a farm. One afternoon a group of chosen kids were to meet at the sheep shed. There were two sheep penned inside this shed. The first one was hauled out in front of everyone as the farmer explained how to shear a sheep, then went on to demonstrate. The sheep looked uncomfortable as it was contortioned into various positions and roughly handled. It was difficult to watch. We stopped for afternoon tea and were told upon our return we would watch the slaughter of this beautiful sentient animal that remained penned up. It had no idea what was about to happen.

I begged not to watch, however was forced to stand behind a wall where I heard everything including feeling the vibration on the rickety floorboards as it kicked and protested until its last breath left its body! I was then made to go sit with the other children as we watched it being strung upside down and the mutilation began. I was ten!

What people don't realise is you can't 'LOVE' animals and eat them. It's in direct conflict. To eat an animal, you are saying it's ok to torture, maim, mutilate, dismember and kill, without regard to the fact that this animal wants to live with every inch of its body, as much as you and I do.

At the dinner table my mum would make exceptions for me and give me tiny morsels of meat that I would try and get down while the family would chomp down steaks and other cuts of meat that I couldn't stand. My mum persisted feeding me meat at mealtimes and even used to make lamb's fry and bacon before netball matches believing it would give me lots of energy to play, YUK!

When I was 17 years old she gave up, and so began my life as a vegetarian.

I never looked back and had never felt better. I researched farming practices, slaughterhouse practices, watched animals getting mutilated without anaesthetic and knew immediately I was doing the right thing, and my convictions strengthened. This continued for many years until I was very excited one November to find out there was a 'World Vegan Day'. I packed my family up and off we went to hang out with other like-minded people… What I was met with was completely unexpected. I wondered what kind of hole I had been living in and became very angry at myself. I had only focused on meat and didn't think how I got my dairy or the treatment of the chickens that laid my eggs. I learnt so much that day about cosmetic testing, the horseracing industry, dairy industry, factory farming, egg laying hens, fur industry and the list goes on. I was so angry with myself that I didn't know these heinous processes were taking place – or did I choose not to know? Seeing the visuals was very confronting and I felt a deep sense of remorse because my continued consumption of dairy and eggs was hurting these beautiful, gentle-natured animals – I haven't eaten these things since and there began my life as a vegan…

To Close Your Eyes, Will Not Ease Anothers Pain

Ancient Chinese Proverb

FRUCTOSE MALABSORPTION

Fructose is a sugar found in a variety of different foods such as grains, fruit, vegetables and natural sweeteners.

Fructose is also found in different forms, such as on its own as a free sugar or bound to each other, forming fructans.

In fructose malabsorption, the sufferer has an inability to absorb the 'excess free fructose' (over and above the glucose levels) and as a result as it enters the large bowel, and the bacterial action rapidly ferments it, causing bloating, tummy rumblings, flatulence, abdominal pain, diarrhoea and/or constipation and urgency.

The symptoms are characteristic of irritable bowel syndrome. One in three IBS sufferers are said to suffer from fructose malabsorption.

Most people can tolerate an upper limit of fructose of approximately 50gm. Those with fructose malabsorption struggle with an upper limit of 25gm.

Symptoms can be managed effectively by avoiding high fructose foods and following a low FODMAP diet.

FODMAPs are a family of carbohydrates that have been found to be problematic for those with fructose malabsorption due to poor assimilation and absorption.

FODMAP is an acronym coined by the researchers at Monash University for fermentable oligosaccharides, disaccharides, monosaccharides and polyols.

Fructose malabsorption can be identified by a simple non-invasive hydrogen breath test.

A nutritionist/dietitian may put the client on an elimination diet post diagnosis for six to eight weeks and then slowly introduce the problematic foods. This will establish tolerance levels and assist the client to better understand the diet. Unlike coeliac disease, there is no damage occurring to the lining of the bowel, just the uncomfortable symptoms the client experiences until the food is eliminated.

MONOSACCHARIDES	DISACCHARIDES	OLIGOSACCHARIDES	POLYOLS
These are free forms of fructose and become problematic when found in higher levels than the glucose content of certain foods.	Commonly lactose, it is two sugar molecules bound together. Lactose is found in dairy products only.	These include fructans and galacto-oligosaccharides and are made up of many 'sugars' joined together making a longer chain.	These are a family of sugar alcohols that include xylitol, erythritol, maltitol, mannitol, sorbitol.
These are found in foods such as honey, apples, agave nectar, pears, watermelon, asparagus, peas, cherries and some fruit juices.	Foods containing lactose include cream, ice cream, milk, yoghurt and custard. Some cheeses have been found to be safe due to the bacterial action on the lactose itself. For further information, please consult your nutritionist/dietitian.	Foods containing these saccharides include legumes, wheat, onion, garlic, rye and couscous.	They are found in foods such as plums, peaches, nectarines, mushrooms, cauliflower, apples and pears, cashews and pistachios.

Due to the increased risk of malnutrition, if you suspect or are diagnosed with fructose malabsorption, it is highly recommended you seek the advice of a professional nutritionist or dietitian.

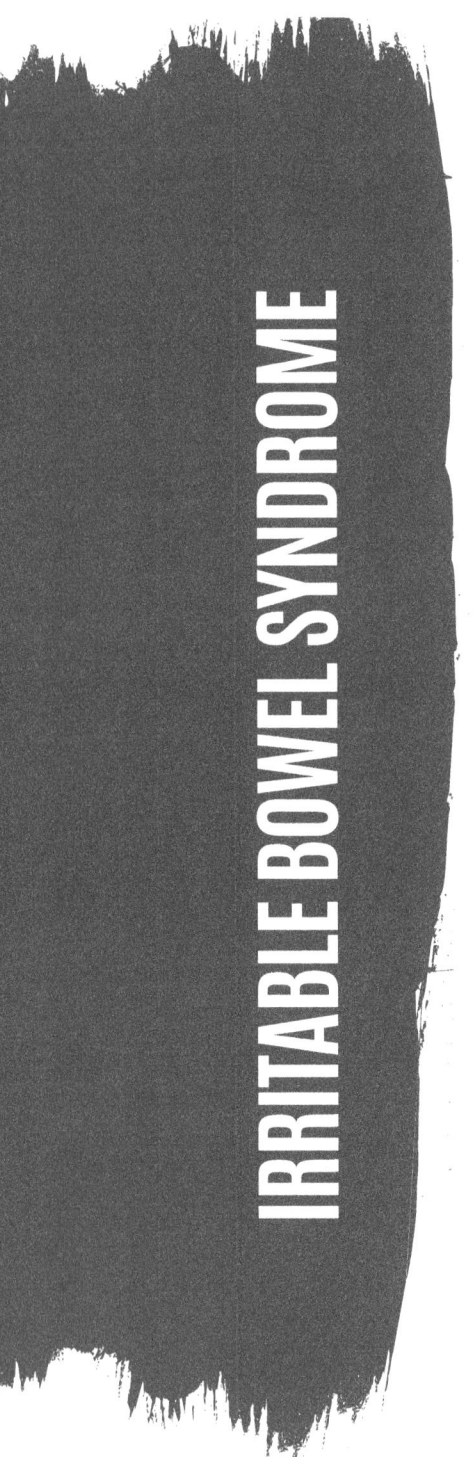

IRRITABLE BOWEL SYNDROME

Irritable bowel syndrome (IBS), according to monashfodmap.com (2021) affects one in seven people. The symptoms include diarrhoea, constipation or a combination or both, abdominal distension, urgency to defecate, abdominal pain, bloating and or excessive wind. Sufferers may also feel fatigued due to the pain in their gut.

There are several potential causes of IBS which can include stress and anxiety, diet, infections, altered levels of good/bad gut bacteria and sensitivity.

Prospective dietary triggers may include but not be exclusive to are:
- High fat diet
- Stimulants such a caffeine, spicy food and laxatives
- Alcohol
- Lactose
- Gluten

According to the Monash University Gastrointestinal dept, it has been noted that 75% of those suffering from IBS and adopted a low FODMAP diet, were better able to manage their symptoms.

If you feel you suffer any of these symptoms please visit your doctor, nutritionist, or dietitian.

COELIAC DISEASE

Coeliac disease (CD) is an autoimmune disease whereby sufferers cannot tolerate gluten. It is estimated that approximately one in seventy Australians have it, however up to 80% remain undiagnosed.

Gluten is a protein found in grains such as wheat, barley, rye, triticale, spelt and kamut. When people with CD come into contact with gluten, it causes inflammation in the small intestine along with antibodies that attack the small hair-like structures that line the intestinal tract called 'villi'. The function of the villi is to increase the surface area of the bowel to optimise absorption of vitamins and minerals. When these structures are damaged, it significantly reduces our ability to absorb nutrients leading to a plethora of deficiency conditions such as poor sleep, gastrointestinal cancers, mood disorders, type 1 diabetes, Addison's disease, amenorrhea, multiple sclerosis, depression, osteoporosis, liver issues, infertility and many more problems.

The most common symptom is diarrhoea. People can also experience bloating, gas, fatigue, anaemia and loss of weight. There is no cure but strict adherence to a gluten free diet sees improvement in symptoms and bowel behaviour.

Diagnosis can only be made via bowel biopsy. If you suffer from any of the said symptoms, please see your doctor.

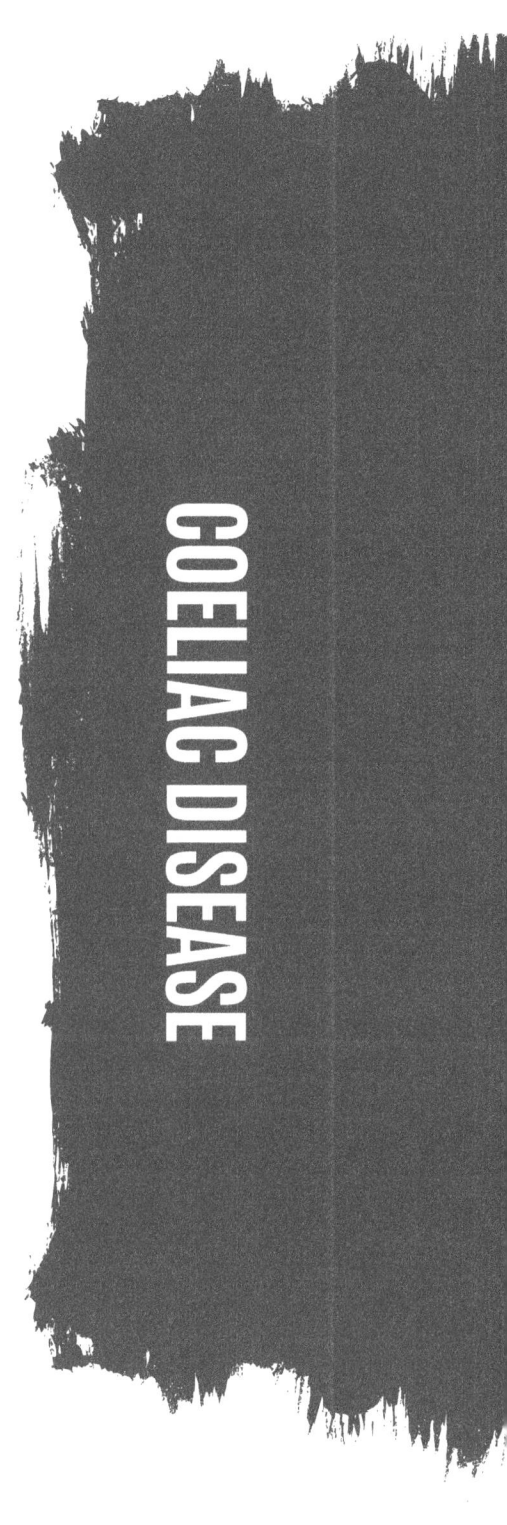

THE PLANTER'S PANTRY

Making a decision to change your health, the health of the planet and decrease cruelty to animals is very exciting and a wonderful beginning on the path to a plant-based diet.

If you are currently eating meat, you must remember this is a journey. If you fall off the wagon and stumble, and consume some meat, don't beat yourself up about it. Get up, shake it off and continue to move forward. Every day you do it, there are fundamental changes that occur within you emotionally and psychologically and it becomes easier and easier until you reach the stage you can't believe you ever ate meat in the first place.

It is a big myth that we need meat and dairy for health, wellbeing, brain development and strong bones and teeth. What we have found through research is, that these foods don't promote but impede health.

To assist you with this journey I have put together some of my favourite pantry staples. This will ensure that you set yourself up for success, to guarantee you maintain your health and don't suffer from deficiencies.

When eating a plant-based diet, you need to eat more to consume your required calories. This is important to note as many people who start their plant-based journey quit prematurely as they start to feel lethargic and fatigued. This is great news for me… you don't have to ask me twice to eat more!

SAVOURY YEAST FLAKES:

One of my all-time favourites, SYF has a delightful nutty, cheesy flavour. It can be eaten raw or cooked, used to make cheese sauces, sprinkle on popcorn or over your favourite steamed vegies. SYF are a complete protein, containing all the B vitamins, iron, selenium and zinc. SYF are also low in fat, low in sodium, are gluten free, sugar free and preservative free. When buying SYF ensure you choose one fortified with vitamin B12. Due to the pasteurisation, this renders the yeast inactive, making them unsuitable for baking but the silver lining is that this makes it safe for those suffering from candida and other yeast infections to still enjoy it.

CHIA SEEDS

Related to the mint family (though doesn't share that distinct minty taste) chia seeds are full of wonderful qualities. They are a complete protein, high in fibre and high in antioxidants. They contain quality amounts of calcium, manganese, magnesium and phosphorous, accompanied by good amounts of zinc, B1, B2, B3 and vitamin K. They are a great source of 'good fats', with a 30gm (2tbs) serve containing 9gm fat of which 5gm are omega~3 (www.healthline.com). Chia seeds are very versatile as they can be used in smoothies, egg replacing or used as a binding agent.

HEMP SEEDS/OIL

Another great plant based complete protein, hemp seeds are rich in omega-3, omega-6, Vitamin E, K and the minerals phosphorous, potassium, sodium, magnesium, calcium, iron and zinc. They can be consumed raw, cooked or toasted and the hearts have a lovely soft nutty flavour. Hemp seeds are 25% protein, which compares favourably to that of beef and lamb. Hemp seeds are also rich in arginine and methionine, two amino acids that can be found lacking in a vegetarian diet.

RAW NUTS – WALNUTS/BRAZIL

One of my favourite foods to snack on. Raw nuts collectively contain a plethora of vitamins, minerals, protein, dietary fibre and good fats. Only two Brazil nuts a day gives you your RDI for selenium (nutritionaustralia.org, viewed 24th September 2017) a mineral found depleted in our over farmed soil grown vegetables. A 30gm serve is all you need, you can eat them straight out of your hand, sprinkle on cereal, through stir fries or add to a homemade trail mix.

WHOLEGRAINS

Rich in dietary fibre, B vitamins, magnesium, iron, selenium, protein and good fats, wholegrains provide a variety of important health benefits from digestive health, heart health, assisting in weight control and making you feel fuller for longer post eating. These include brown rice, millet, amaranth and quinoa. Unless you have coeliac disease, gluten intolerance or other medical cause for avoiding certain grains, enjoy them in a variety of ways from porridge, pilaf, salads and the list goes on.

RICEMALT SYRUP/MAPLE SYRUP

These are a great replacement for sweeteners, with maple being quite a bit sweeter that rice malt syrup. Maple syrup must be 100% pure and not maple flavoured. They are gluten free, fructose free and low FODMAP. They can be used in baking, on pancakes or whatever else you would use honey for.

COCONUT MILK/CREAM/OIL

Anything from a coconut is so versatile. Used in small amounts the milk and cream can be used in curries, desserts and making ice cream. The oil can be used to fry foods due to its high heat tolerance. It is also antibacterial and antifungal making it a great addition to the pantry. They contain good fats that supports weight control and blood sugar control.

CINNAMON

Used in both savoury and sweet dishes I love this little gem. Cinnamon has so many health-giving properties including being used as a natural preserver. It aids to balance blood sugar levels and is antiviral, antibacterial and antifungal. Cinnamon is also a great antioxidant and anti-inflammatory, so a great addition to the pantry. Ceylon is considered 'true cinnamon' as it has lower levels of the compound coumarin. Cassia contains high levels, which can cause problems in large doses – if using cassia try to limit it to 1–2 tsp daily.

TAHINI

Rich in nutrients, this is one of the best sources of plant-based calcium with 15gm giving 64mg calcium. It is also rich in vitamin E, B's, K and magnesium. With so many uses such as adding it to salad dressing, binding bliss balls, adding to avocado to enhance your 'smash' or blending with chickpeas to make hummus, tahini has a place in everyone's pantry. Keep your serving moderate to maintain desirable levels.

SEA VEGETABLES

Sea vegetables are rich in iodine – a nutrient often found lacking in the plant-based diet. Examples of sea vegies like nori, arame and dulse contain quality amounts of Vitamin C, manganese, B2 and many other trace vitamins and minerals. They can be consumed in a variety of ways such as added to soups, salads, wrapped as a sushi roll and vegie dishes.

LEGUMES

Canned lentils and a small amount of canned chickpeas is a must for any vego pantry ensuring the quantities stay within threshold limits. They are high in protein, dietary fibre, and Vitamin B complex. In fact, one cup of lentils provides you with 90% of your daily needs of folate (adult). Beans are also a great mineral source with one cup of lentils providing 37% of your daily iron needs (adult). Beans have had a bad rap at times due to their phytic acid levels. Phytic acid binds to minerals making them unavailable for our bodies to absorb. They also contain the antinutrient, lectin. These resist digestion and can at times damage the lining of the gastrointestinal tract. There is hope though. By soaking, sprouting or fermenting the legumes, we break down these antinutrients making nutrients more bioavailable. This is great news as legumes aid in weight loss, heart health and stabilising our blood sugar.

MISO

Made from fermented beans and certain grains, miso has been traditionally used to treat various complaints, those including digestive upsets and to relieve inflammation. Miso contains trace amounts of copper, magnesium, potassium, zinc, phosphorous and choline. Per tablespoon it contains 2gm protein and is only 34 calories. What it is best known for is it teems with beneficial live bacteria. These enter our gut environment and out balance the 'bad' bacteria helping to support digestion and improve our immune system. It can be used to make dressing for salads, vegetables, tofu, added to stir fries or as I like to drink it like a 'cup of soup'. Adding one teaspoon to hot water and 1 teaspoon of sea vegies. Let is sit until sea vegies are soft and enjoy. If you are gluten intolerant, ensure to check ingredient lists prior to purchase as it can be made from gluten containing grains.

TOFU/TEMPEH

Tempeh is made from fermented soybeans and yields more than 50% the protein of tofu, equalling 18gm per 100gm. Along with this, tempeh contains great levels of vitamins B2, B3, B5 and B6. As any fermented food, it is rich with lifegiving bacteria supporting gut and immune health. Tofu also contains all the amino acids and is an excellent source of iron and calcium. Ensure when purchasing these products that you check it is not made from GM produce. Tofu and tempeh are so versatile. They can be used as sandwich fillings, stir fries, curries, desserts. I love to thinly slice firm tofu and place in a hot fry pan with some tamari and cook until it's crispy. It comes out chewy and salty and is great in a TLT (TLT – tofu, lettuce and tomato) or a Caesar salad. Avoid silken tofu if sensitive to it.

SEEDS

Pumpkin seeds, flax seeds, sesame seeds and sunflower seeds are a great addition to so many dishes. Add them to trail mixes – mixing them with your raw nuts and dried fruits for a rich energy giving snack. Add them to bliss balls, throw them in a stir fry, grind and add to baking, add to muesli bars and they add a great crunch to salads. Collectively, these guys provide good fats, zinc, calcium, iron, vitamin E, protein, magnesium, and are beautifully rich in B vitamins. We don't break down whole flaxseeds very efficiently so if not soaking them for digestive purposes, it is always a great idea to grind them first.

RAW APPLE CIDER VINEGAR

With its numerous health benefits, ACV is rich in potassium, acetic acid, magnesium, probiotics and enzymes. It is a great kickstart to any day. I begin my day with a glass of filtered water, 1 tbs ACV, pinch of Himalayan sea salt, pinch of cayenne and the juice of ½ a lemon. When purchasing ACV ensure it has not been pasteurised or filtered. You want it with the floaty bits – 'the Mother'. The Mother contains all those delicious digestive enzymes and probiotics.

EAT A RAINBOW

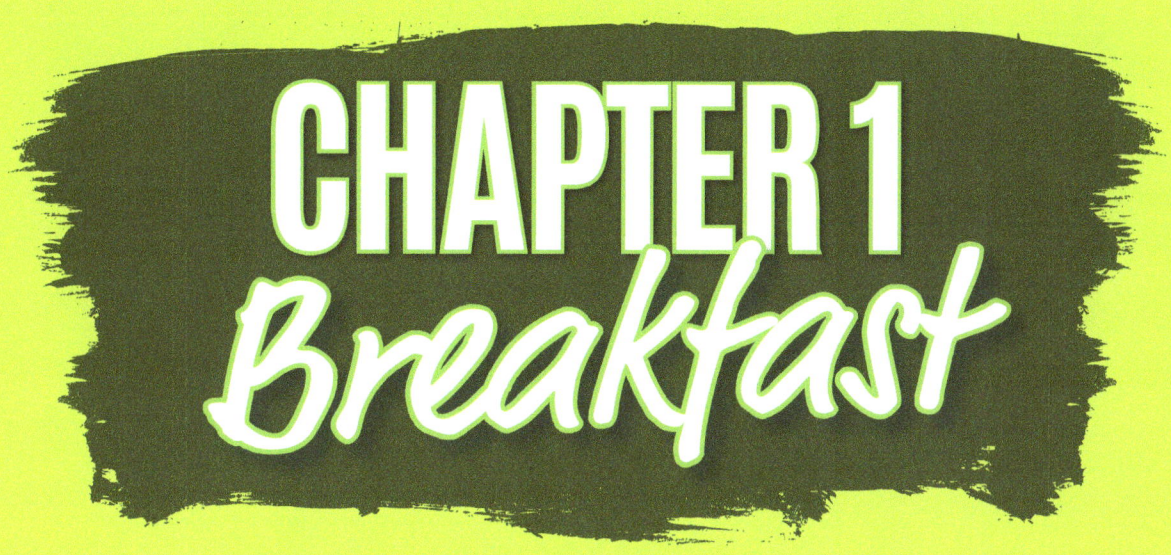

CHAPTER 1
Breakfast

"If we could live happy and healthy lives without harming others, why wouldn't we?"

– Pam Ahern, Edgars Mission

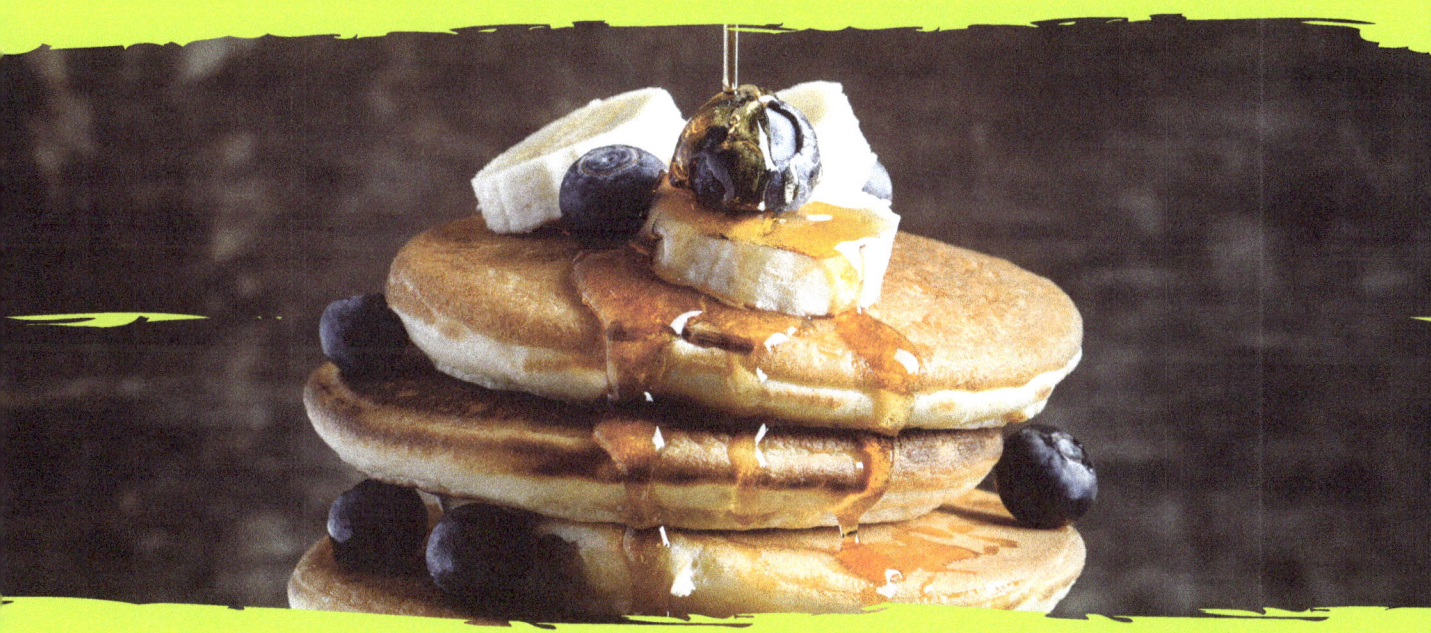

Breakfast is traditionally the most important meal of the day. After 'fasting' all night, you are considered to be breaking the 'FAST' when you rise and consume your first meal of the day.

It is recommended you start your day with a glass of filtered water with fresh lemon juice. Approximately 20 minutes later you can enjoy your breakfast.

As most of us would not have eaten for about six to eight hours, it is important to start your day off correctly with a hearty, fibre rich and sustaining meal. This can vary from the Saturday morning cook up, porridge or greens on grainy toast. YUM…

SCRAMBLED TOFU

This is one of my all-time favourite breakfasts. It is quick, nutritious, tasty and really filling. The turmeric aids to reduce inflammation and the tofu is rich in calcium and protein. A great start to any day.

PREPARATION TIME
20 MINUTES

COOKING TIME
15 MINUTES

SERVES
4

INGREDIENTS:

350gm tofu firm, non-GMO
80ml plant-based milk of your choice
10gm turmeric
5gm kala namak
2 medium carrots
2 spring onions, green parts only
5 stalks parsley finely chopped
30ml garlic infused oil
Himalayan sea salt and black pepper to taste

METHOD:

1. Wash tofu and crumble it into a bowl.
2. Add plant milk, turmeric and black salt, blend and set aside.
3. Peel and grate carrots.
4. Chop the green parts of the spring onions.
5. Heat oil in a large fry pan.
6. Add carrots, zucchini and spring onions, stirring and frying until they wilt.
7. Add tofu mix and blend thoroughly. Cook for about 5 minutes constantly stirring so as it doesn't stick.
8. Just before serving, add the parsley, reserving some florets for the garnish.
9. Season with Himalayan sea salt and black pepper to taste.

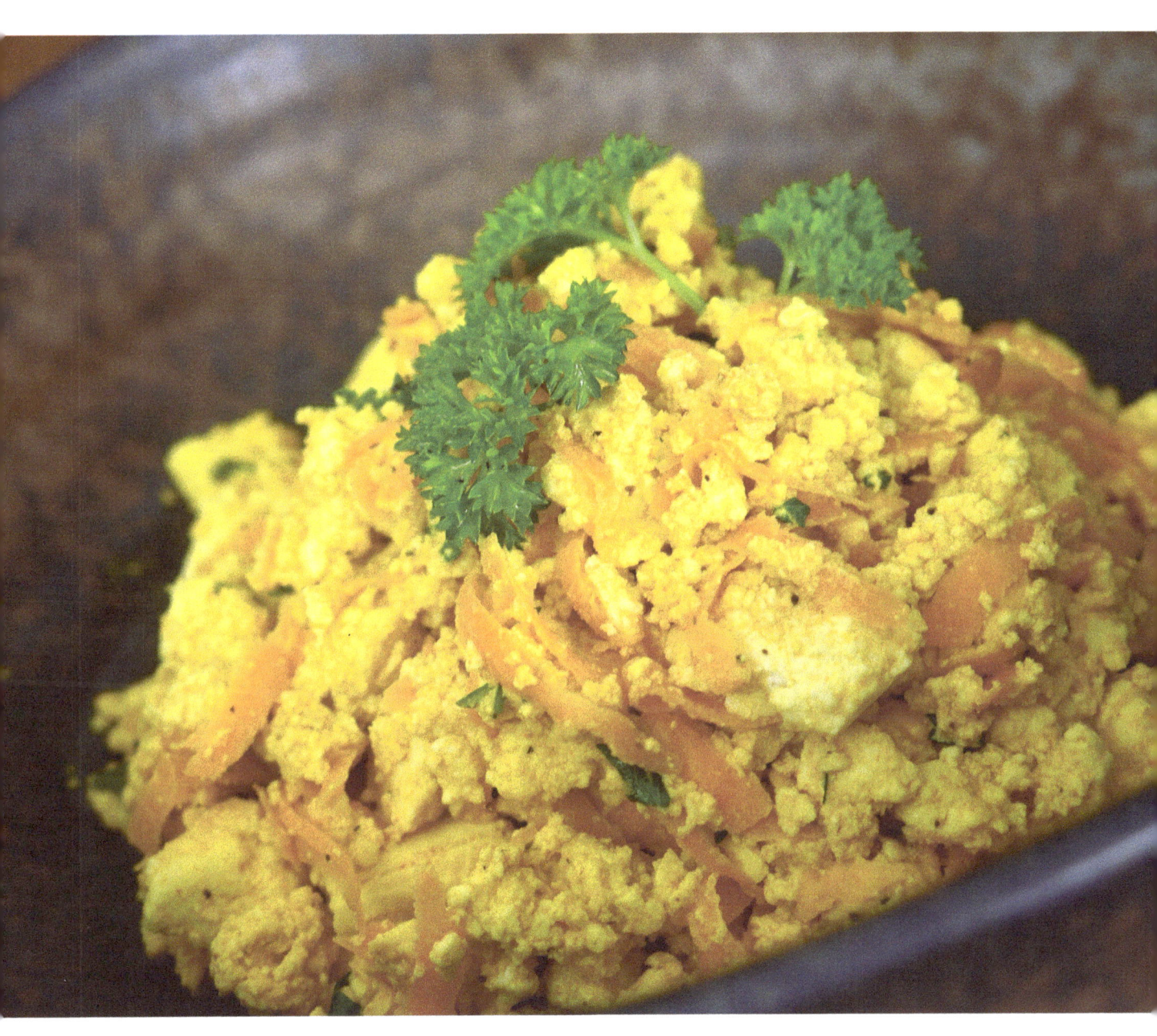

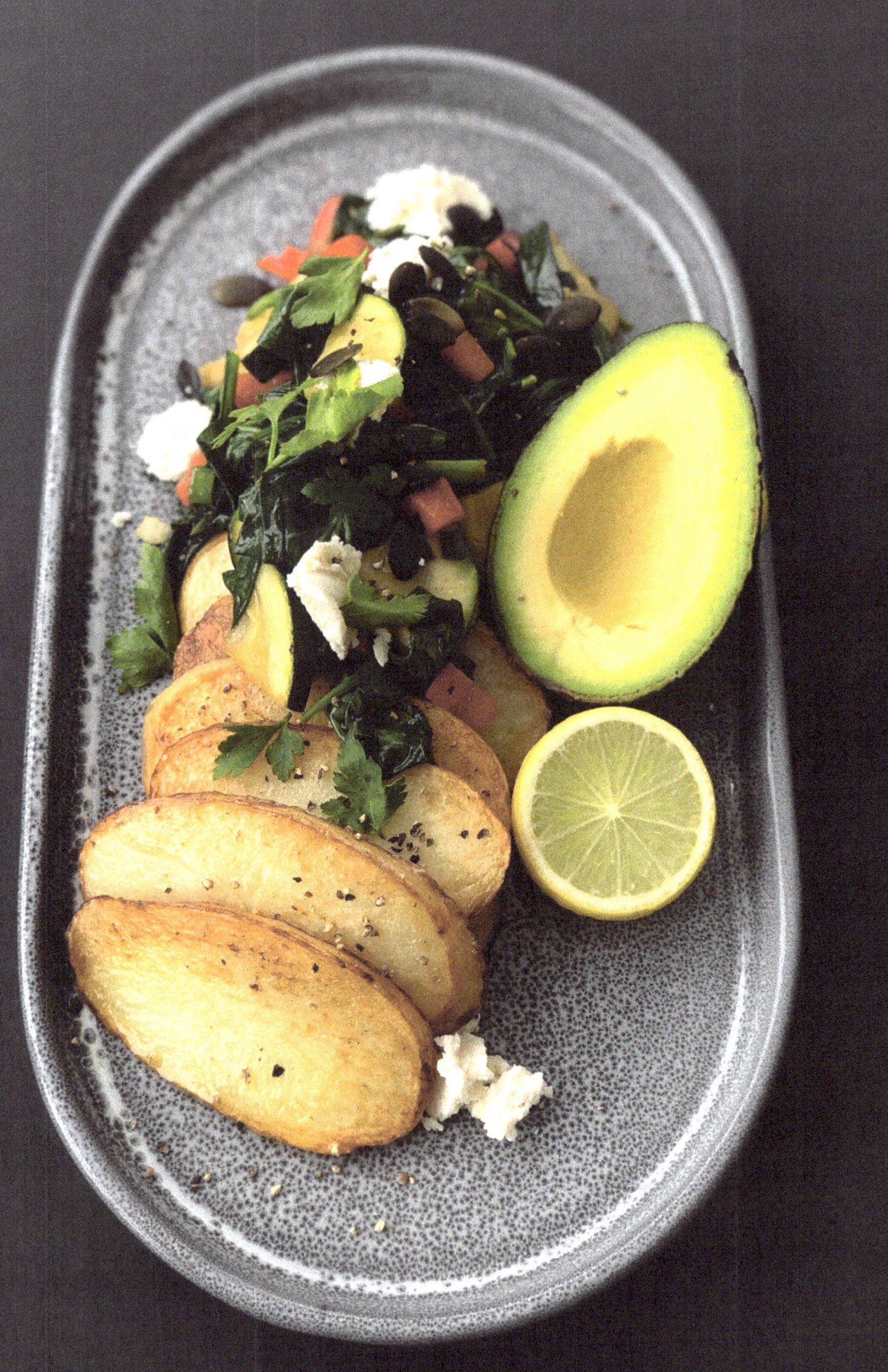

BIG BREAKY

Who doesn't love a big breaky on that lazy day off? We make this regularly on the weekends and is a favourite day starter. Full of vitamins and minerals, you can be sure you are starting your day off right.

PREPARATION TIME
15 MINUTES

COOKING TIME
20 MINUTES

SERVES
3

INGREDIENTS:

Garlic infused oil
3 medium potatoes washed and unpeeled
3 spring onions – green parts only
1 leek, green part only
1 small zucchini
½ red capsicum
2 handfuls baby spinach
½ avocado
5 stalks of parsley
½ lemon
Himalayan sea salt and black pepper to taste
Macadamia feta to serve
20gm pepitas to serve

METHOD:

1. Wash and slice potatoes thinly.
2. Heat oil in a fry pan and add potatoes, cooking them until browned. Once cooked on both sides, set aside.
3. Slice zucchini, finely slice spring onions, greens of the leek and dice capsicum. Add to the hot fry pan the potatoes were cooked in. Add a pinch of salt and cook until softened.
4. Once vegetables have cooked, take off the heat and add 2 handfuls of baby spinach, gently stir until just wilted.
5. Add diced avocado and toss lightly.
6. Place potatoes on serving plate, top with the vegetables.
7. Drizzle with lemon juice and sprinkle pepitas and crumbled feta, season to taste.

BANANA PANCAKES

Bananas are one of my favourite fruits. They come in their own protective packaging and provide potassium for the heart and tryptophan and B6 for good mood.

PREPARATION TIME
15 MINUTES

COOKING TIME
8 MINUTES PER PANCAKE

SERVES
3

INGREDIENTS:

120gm GF wholemeal SR flour
Non-dairy milk
5ml vanilla essence
2 bananas
20gm flaxseed meal
Vegan margarine
½ lemon juiced
100% maple syrup – for serving
Fresh berries for serving

METHOD:

1. Place flour and linseed meal in bowl.
2. Add enough milk to make a nice smooth consistency – not too runny.
3. Add vanilla essence and chopped banana, blend together until just mixed.
4. Melt margarine in a fry pan, place dessert spoons of mix into the fry pan and cook until brown on each side.
5. Drizzle with maple syrup and lemon juice.
6. Serve with fresh berries.

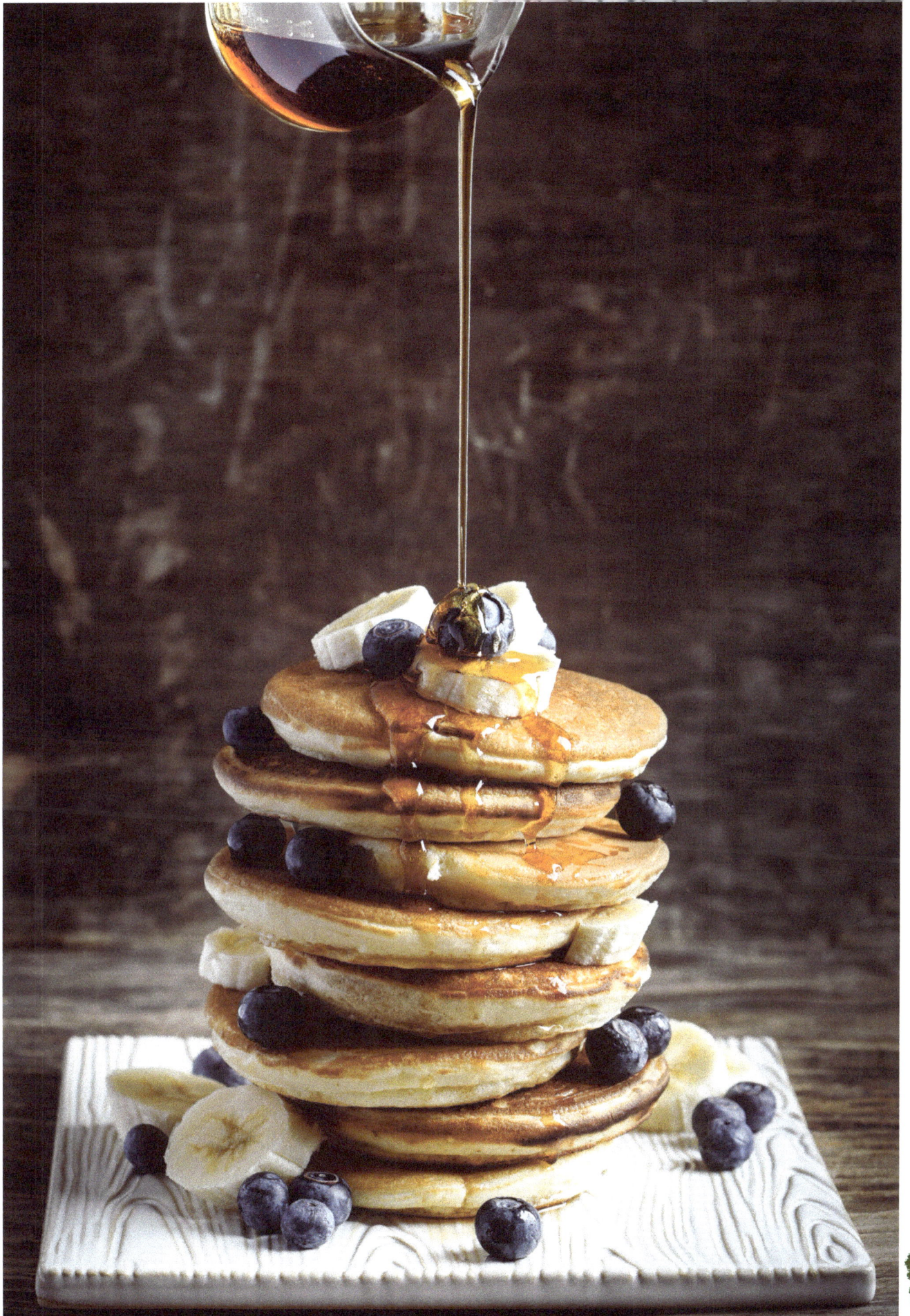

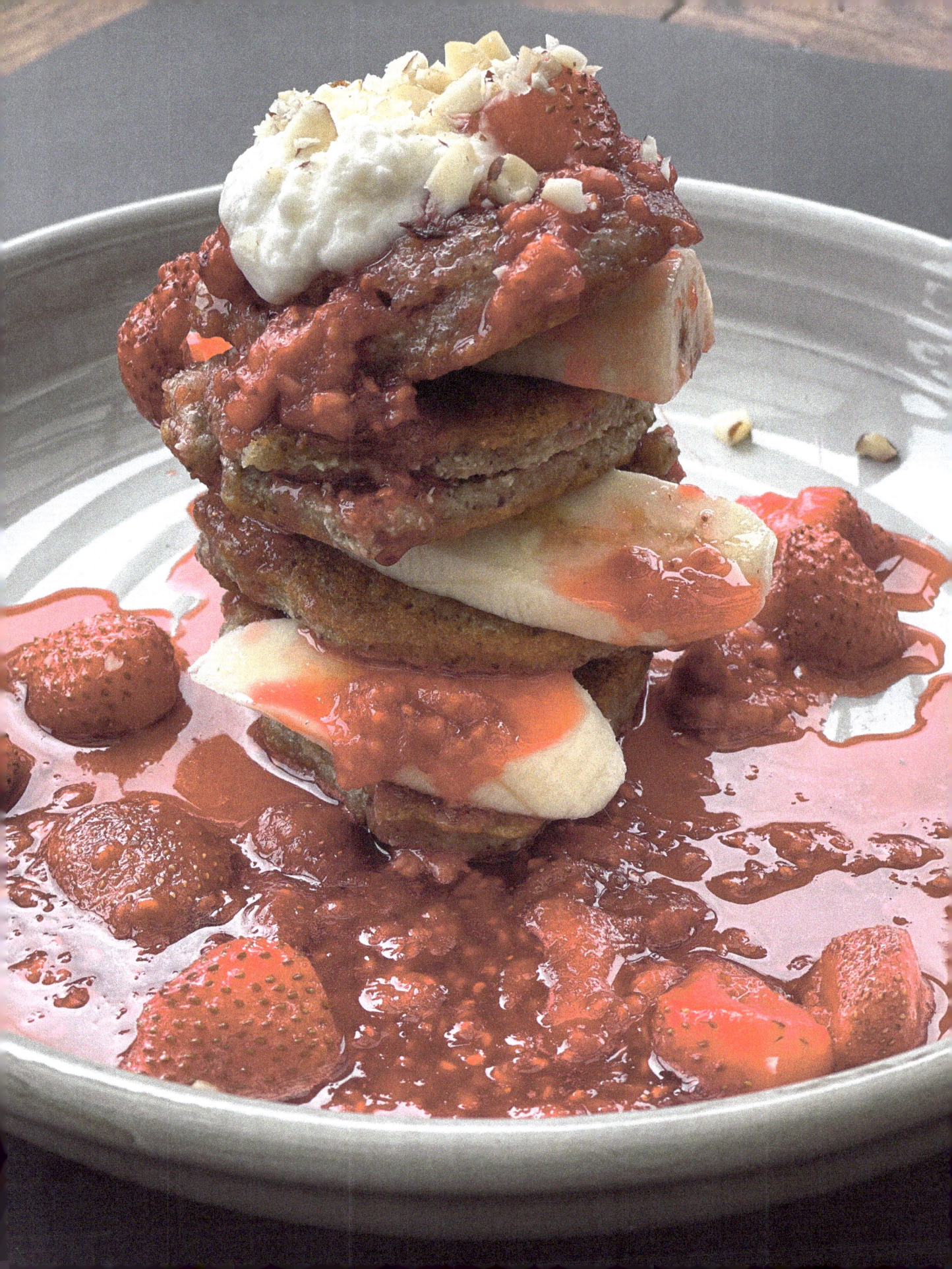

COCONUT FLOUR PANCAKES

PREPARATION TIME
15 MINUTES

COOKING TIME
5 MINUTES

SERVES
3

INGREDIENTS:

30gm coconut flour
125gm GF flour
10gm flaxseed meal
2gm baking soda aluminium free
80ml natural coconut yogurt
1/2 banana
10ml vanilla extract
200ml plant-based milk
Spices of your choosing:
approximately 2gm each cinnamon,
ginger and cardamom
Coconut oil for cooking

METHOD:

1. Mix the flours, flaxseed meal, and baking soda together. Stir and add any spices of choice.

2. In a blender add the non-dairy milk, yogurt, banana, and vanilla extract. Blend thoroughly. If you don't have a blender, you can just combine them in a bowl and use a hand mixer, mashing banana first.

3. Add the dry ingredients to your blended wet ingredients and stir until no lumps can be found.

4. Batter will thicken upon sitting.

5. Coat a medium size fry pan with some coconut oil and place over low-medium heat.

6. Using a tablespoon of the batter at a time, dollop the mixture into the fry pan. Allow it to cook until the bottom edges start to turn golden brown. Carefully flip and cook for one more minute on the other side.

7. Remove from fry pan, place on a plate, and repeat until there is no more batter.

8. Top with coconut yoghurt and your choice of fruit, cocoa nibs, crushed nuts, berry coulis. Whatever takes your mood ☺

This recipe makes enough for 6 pancakes. Halve, double, or even triple it, depending on how many pancakes you want to make. You can also keep these in the freezer in a freezer-safe bag, for on the go breakfasts and snacks. These pancakes are quite heavy, so you really know you have eaten. They keep you full for a long time.

SMOOTHIES

BREAKFAST SMOOTHIE

INGREDIENTS:

500ml non-dairy milk
1 small frozen banana
1.5gm cinnamon
15gm chia seeds
60gm peanut butter

METHOD:

Place all ingredients in blender and blitz until smooth.

GREENS SMOOTHIE

INGREDIENTS:

50ml coconut water
150ml filtered water
1 small handful baby spinach
1 handful chopped kale
150ml pineapple juice
3gm barley grass
3gm spirulina

METHOD:

Place in blender and blitz until smooth. Add more or less of ingredients according to flavour and tolerance levels.

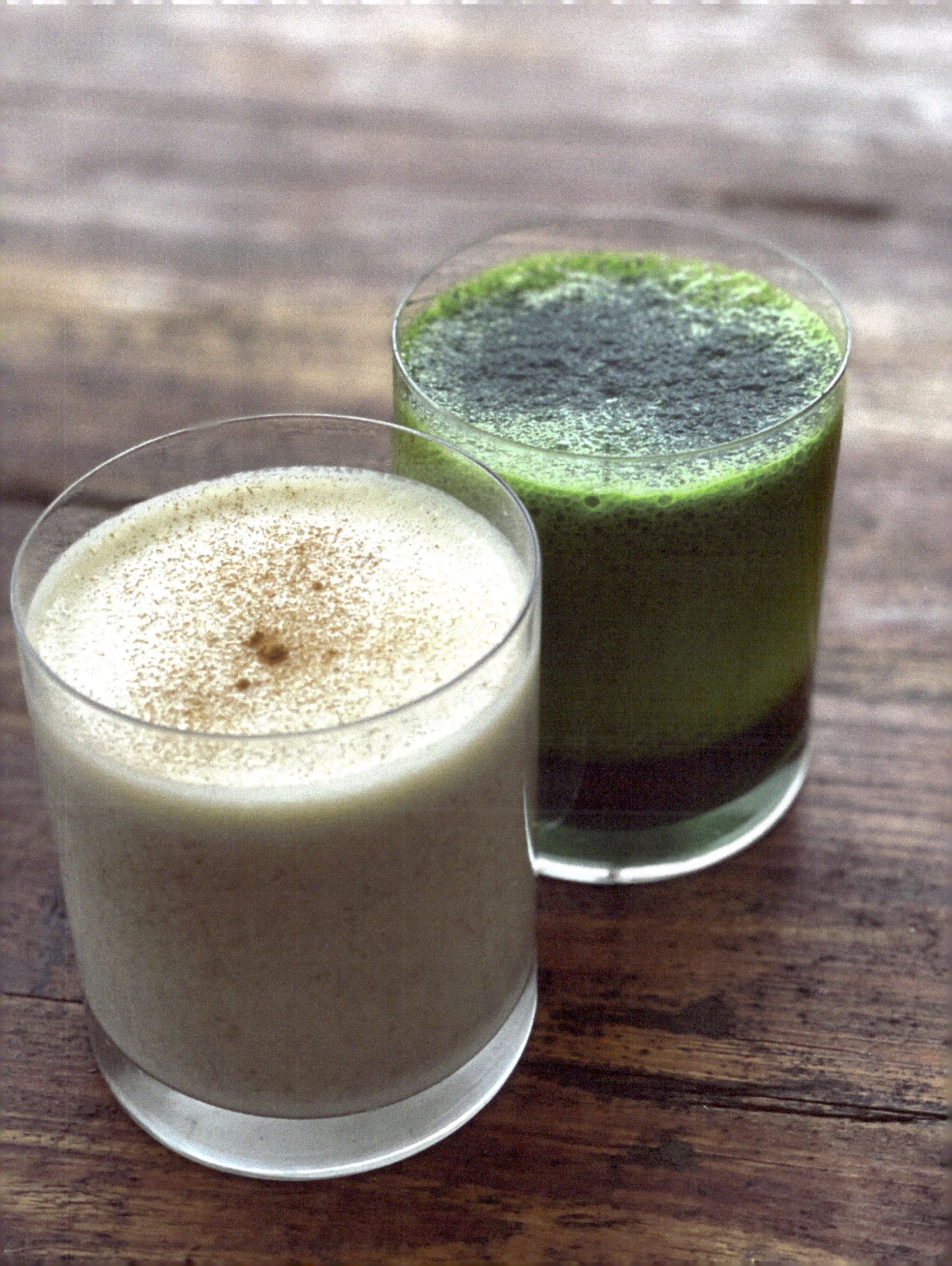

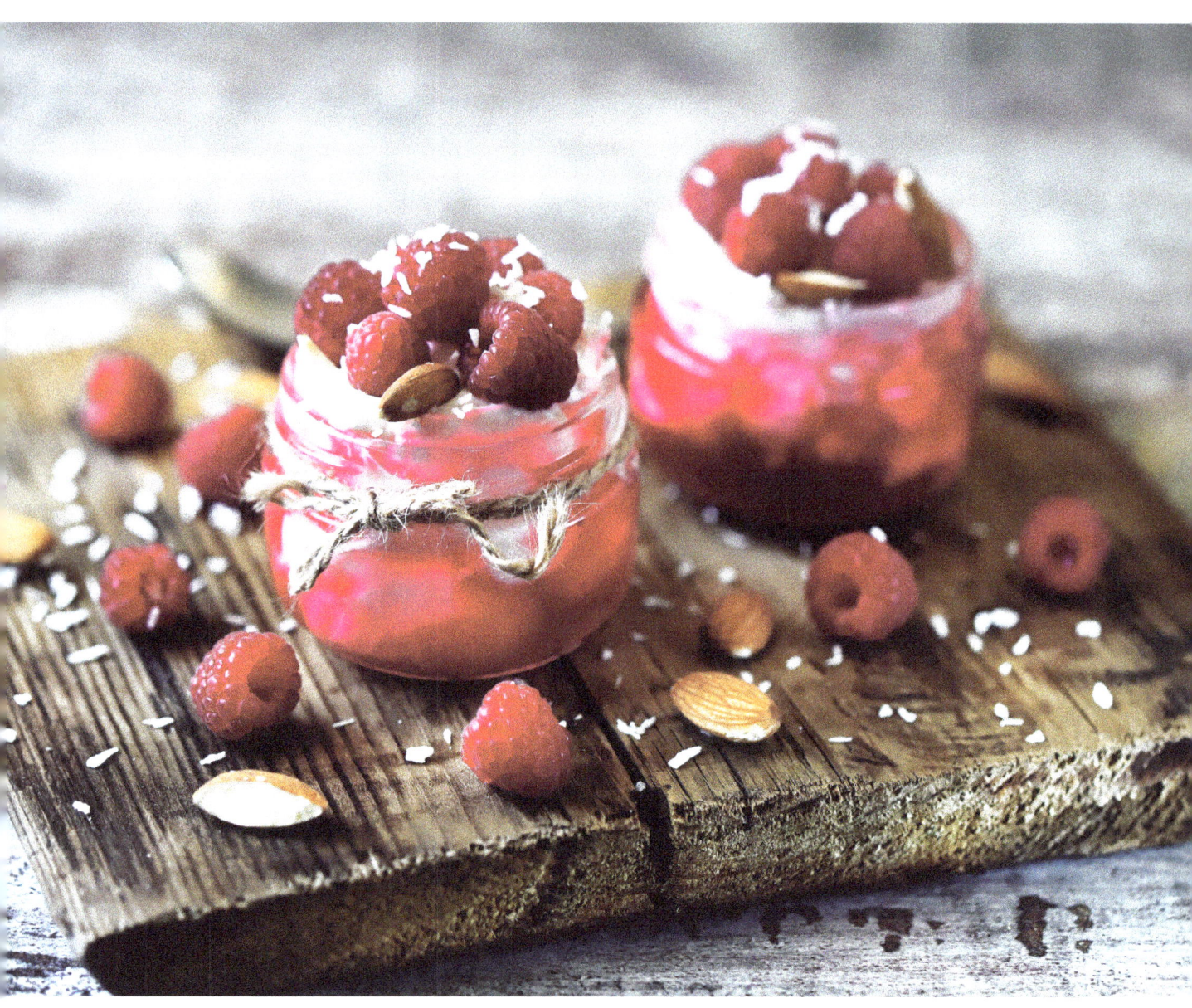

BREAKFAST ON THE GO

Everyone is in such a hurry these days.
This breakfast on the go gives you everything you need to power up for the start of a busy day.

INGREDIENTS:

125gm vanilla coconut yoghurt
5gm flaxseed meal
5 strawberries – more if required
5 raspberries – more if required
½ banana (optional)
½ kiwi fruit (optional)
Sprinkle cinnamon

METHOD:

1. Place yoghurt in a bowl or jar.
2. Sprinkle toppings over the yoghurt and enjoy.

To ensure this remains low FODMAP, bulk up your breakfast with suitable fruits, nuts, GF granola and flaxseed meal.

This can be made the night before, in a jar ready to grab and go.

BREAKFAST BURRITO

PREPARATION TIME
20 MINUTES

COOKING TIME
15 MINUTES

SERVES
8 BURRITOS

INGREDIENTS:

8 GF tortilla wraps
1 batch scrambled tofu
2 tomatoes
2 handfuls baby spinach
3 spring onions, green tops only
1 avocado
Juice ½ lemon
Salt and pepper to taste

METHOD:

1. Preheat oven to 180°C.
2. Slice tomatoes, set aside.
3. Wash and drain spinach.
4. Finely slice spring onions, set aside.
5. Mash avocado with a fork, add lemon juice and season to taste.
6. Turn oven to 150°C.
7. Wrap tortillas in foil and heat in oven until nice and bendy.
8. Spread avocado mix on all 8 tortillas.
9. Spread tofu mix on top of the tortillas.
10. Add sliced tomato, baby spinach and sprinkle with finely sliced spring onions.
11. Season to taste.
12. Wrap them up and enjoy.

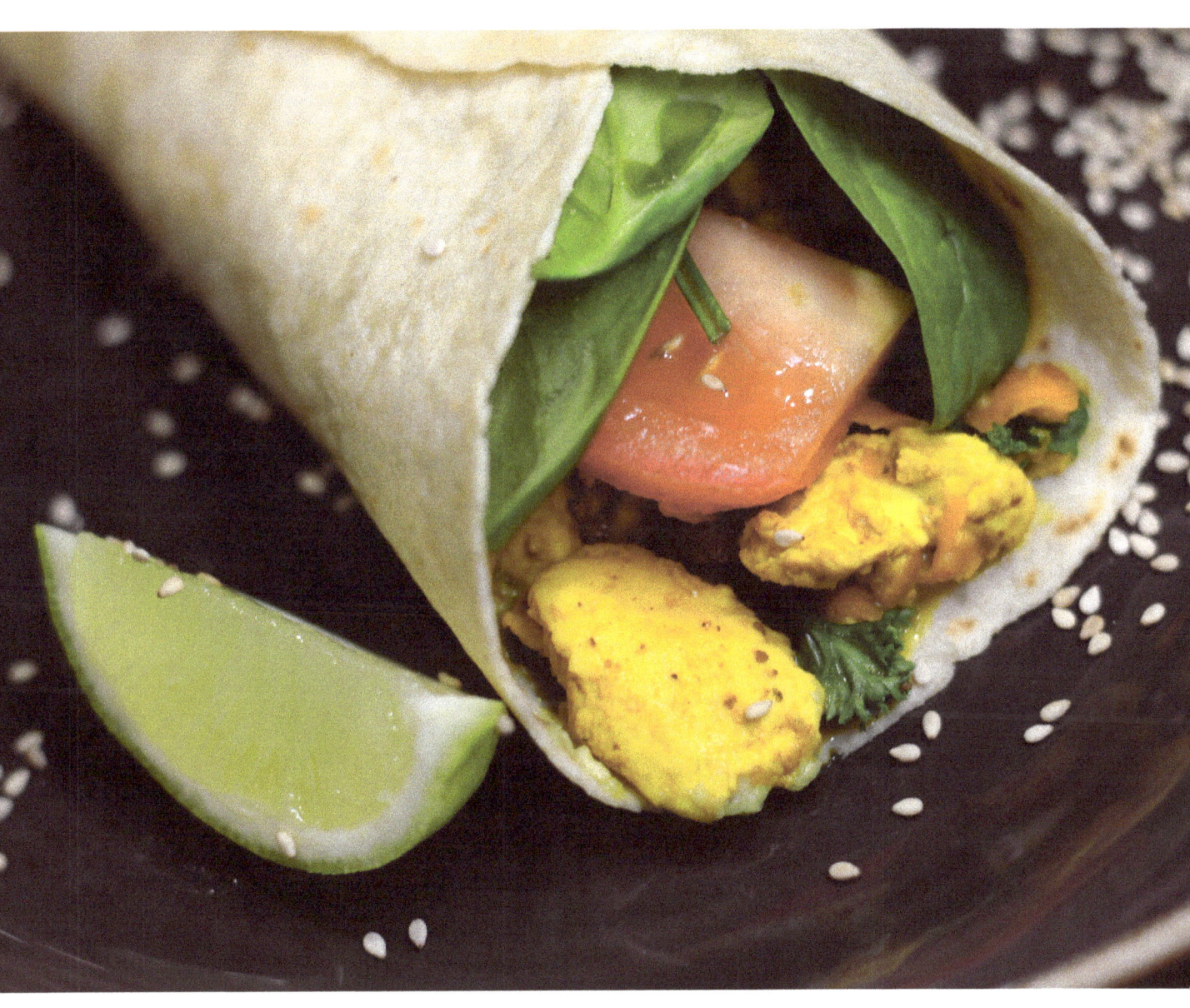

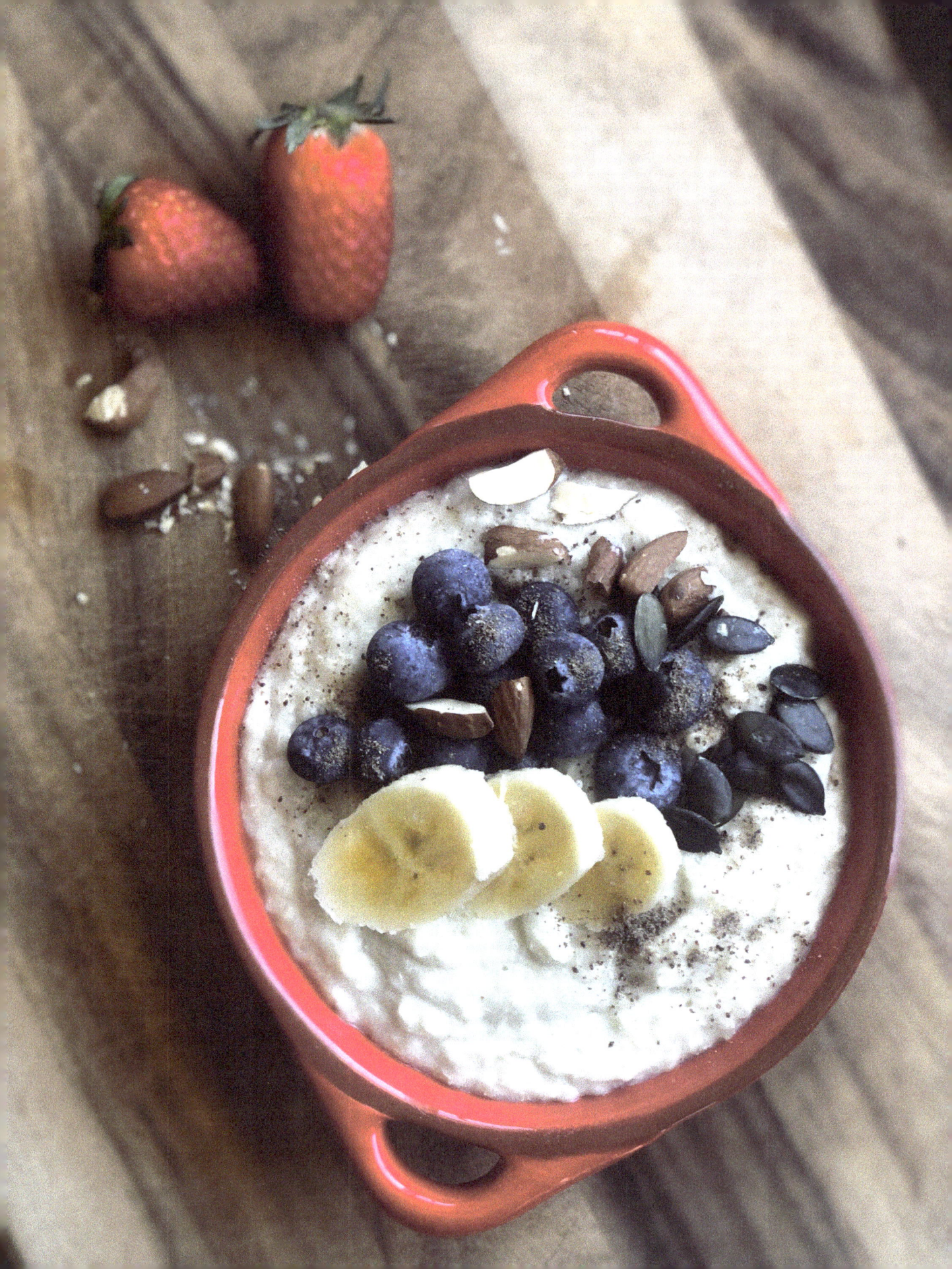

CREAMY QUINOA PORRIDGE

PREPARATION TIME
10 MINUTES

COOKING TIME
10 MINUTES

SERVES
1

INGREDIENTS:

30gm quinoa flakes
125ml water
125ml coconut cream
Pinch Himalayan sea salt
Pinch cinnamon

METHOD:

1. Place quinoa, water, coconut milk, salt and cinnamon into a saucepan.
2. Bring to the boil stirring continuously.
3. Once boiled, let simmer 3 minutes, stirring occasionally.
4. Pour into a bowl, dress with chosen fruit, coconut yoghurt, LSA, pepitas, hemp seeds, berries, sliced banana, nut butter.

VARIATION:

1. Add 5gm raw cocoa to saucepan and cook with the mix.
2. Add 25gm nut butter to saucepan once quinoa is cooked.
3. Add 10gm rice protein powder to saucepan once quinoa is cooked.

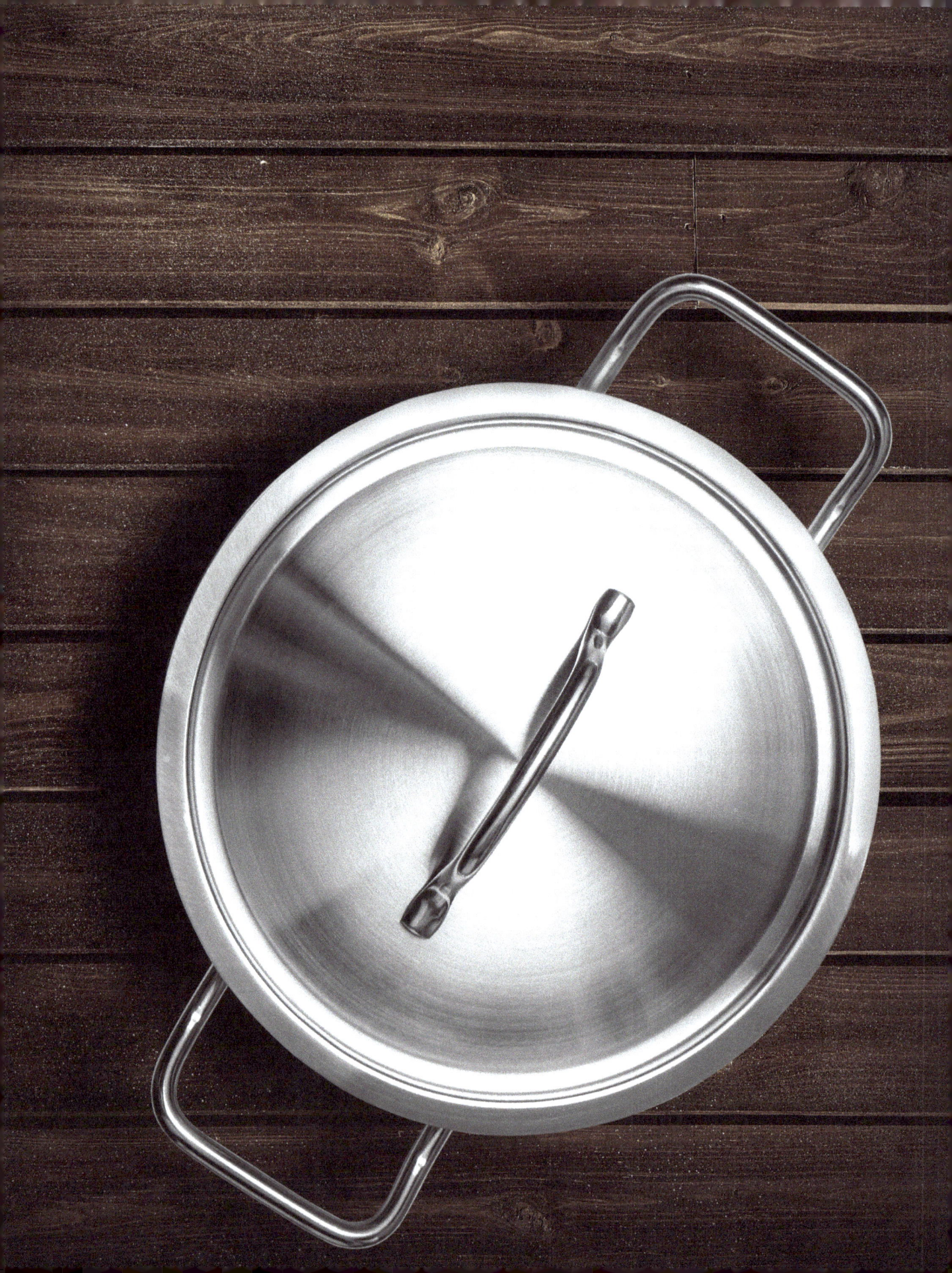

CHAPTER 2
Soups

"It is man's sympathy to all creatures that first makes him truly a man."
— Dr Albert Schweitzer

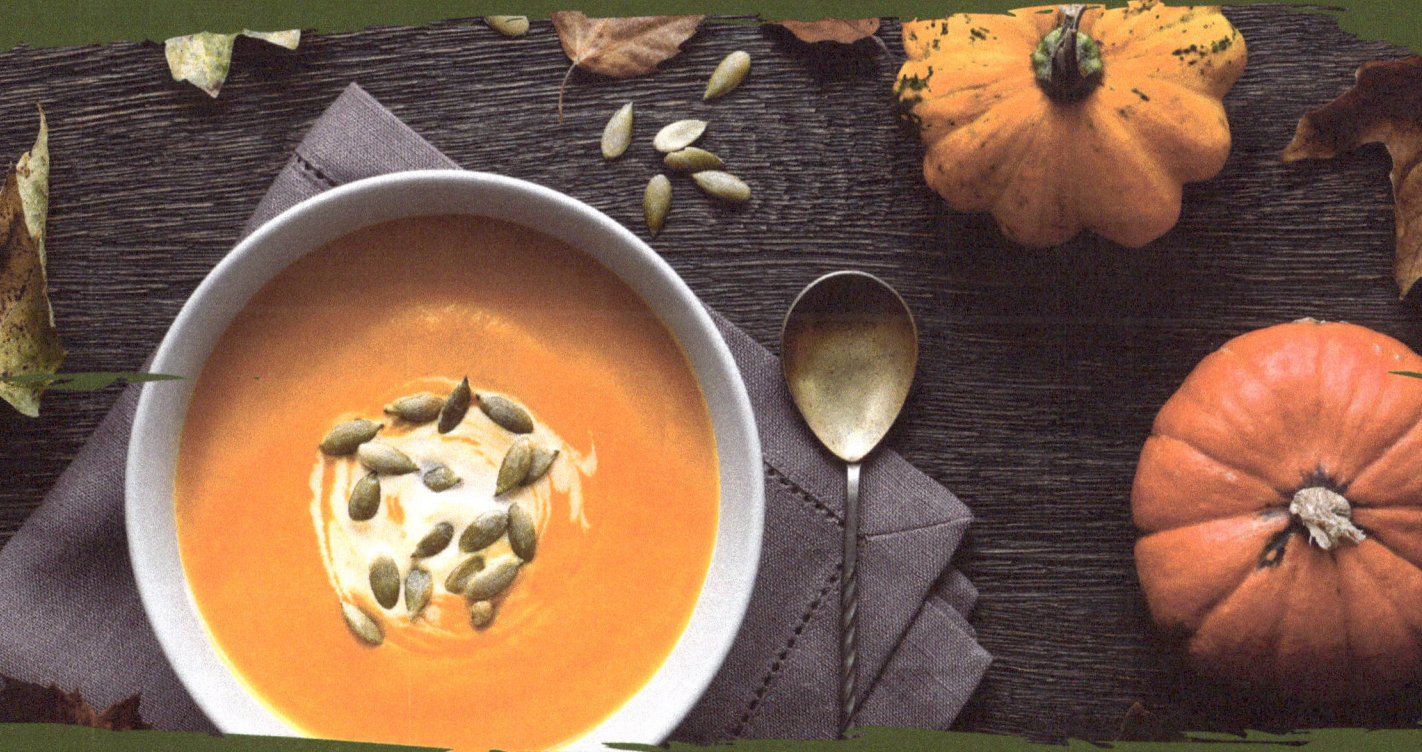

Soups are what I call a 'Nutrient Injection.' I absolutely love them, and they are only limited by your own imagination. You can make a multitude of flavours and varieties, using the amazing produce that our country has to offer, along with gorgeously fresh herbs and spices to elevate and enhance depths of flavour. Hope you enjoy these ones.

BAKED PUMPKIN AND NUTMEG SOUP

PREPARATION TIME
30 MINUTES

COOKING TIME
2 HOURS

SERVES
8

INGREDIENTS:

2.5kg Kent pumpkin
30ml rice bran oil
2.5gm nutmeg
2 stalks celery
1.5kg potatoes
60ml garlic infused oil
2.5l water or low FODMAP vegetable stock
Salt and pepper to taste
Pumpkin seeds – lightly toasted (optional)

METHOD:

1. Preheat oven to 200°C.
2. Peel, deseed and dice pumpkin in approximately 4cm x 4cm size.
3. Toss pumpkin in rice bran oil and place on lined baking tray.
4. Sprinkle with nutmeg and sea salt and bake until golden brown, approximately 30 minutes.
5. Cut celery into approximately 1cm lengths.
6. Heat garlic infused oil in large heavy based saucepan; add celery and sauté until starts to soften.
7. Add roughly chopped potatoes, cooked pumpkin and water (enough to cover).
8. Bring to the boil and then simmer for at least 1.5 hours.
9. Turn off heat and puree with stick blender until smooth. Adjust thickness with additional water or stock to desired texture.
10. Season to taste and serve. For a creamier finish consider adding vegan sour cream and top with toasted pumpkin seeds for crunch.

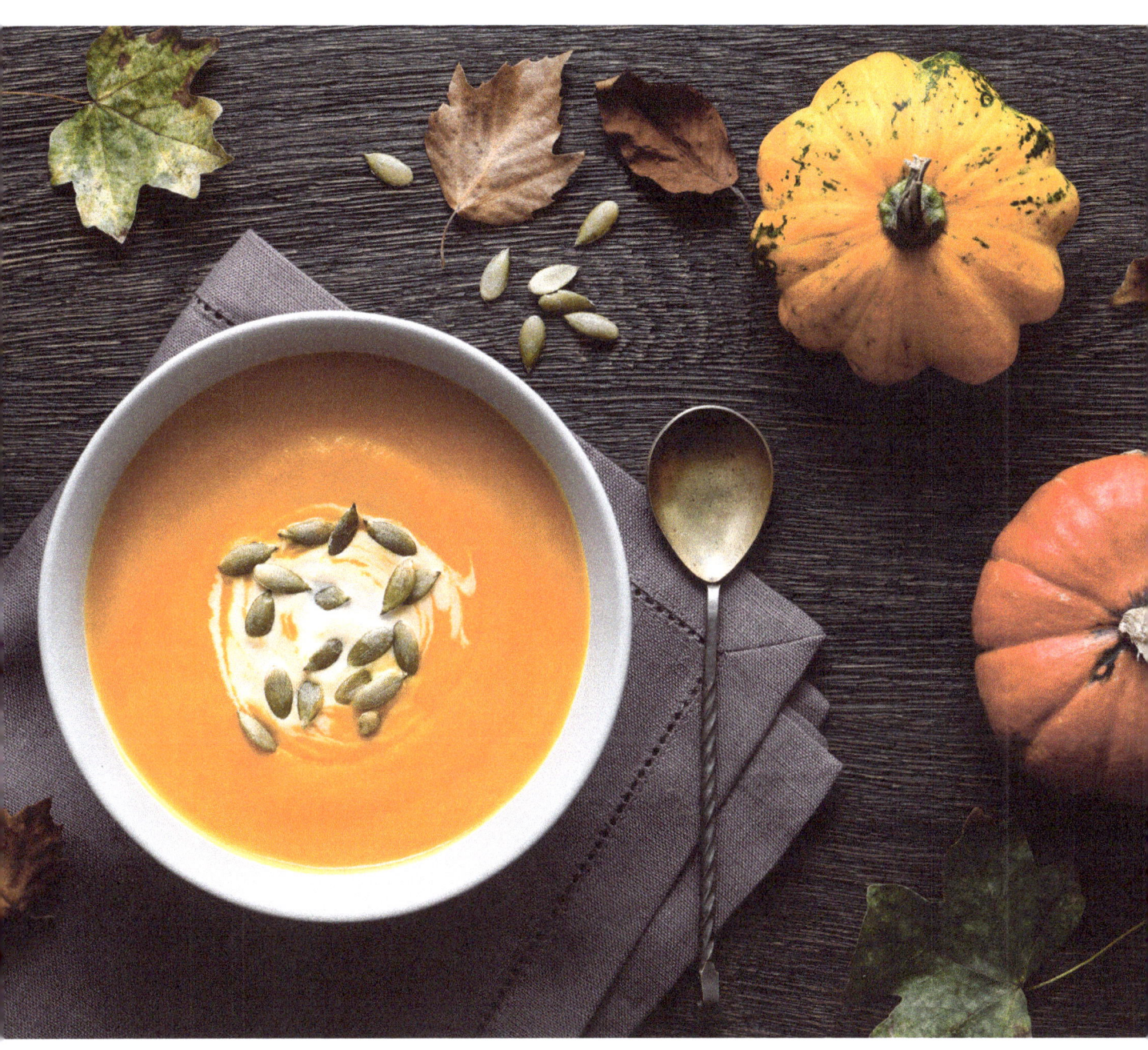

Jodie Martin | **Chapter 2** Soups

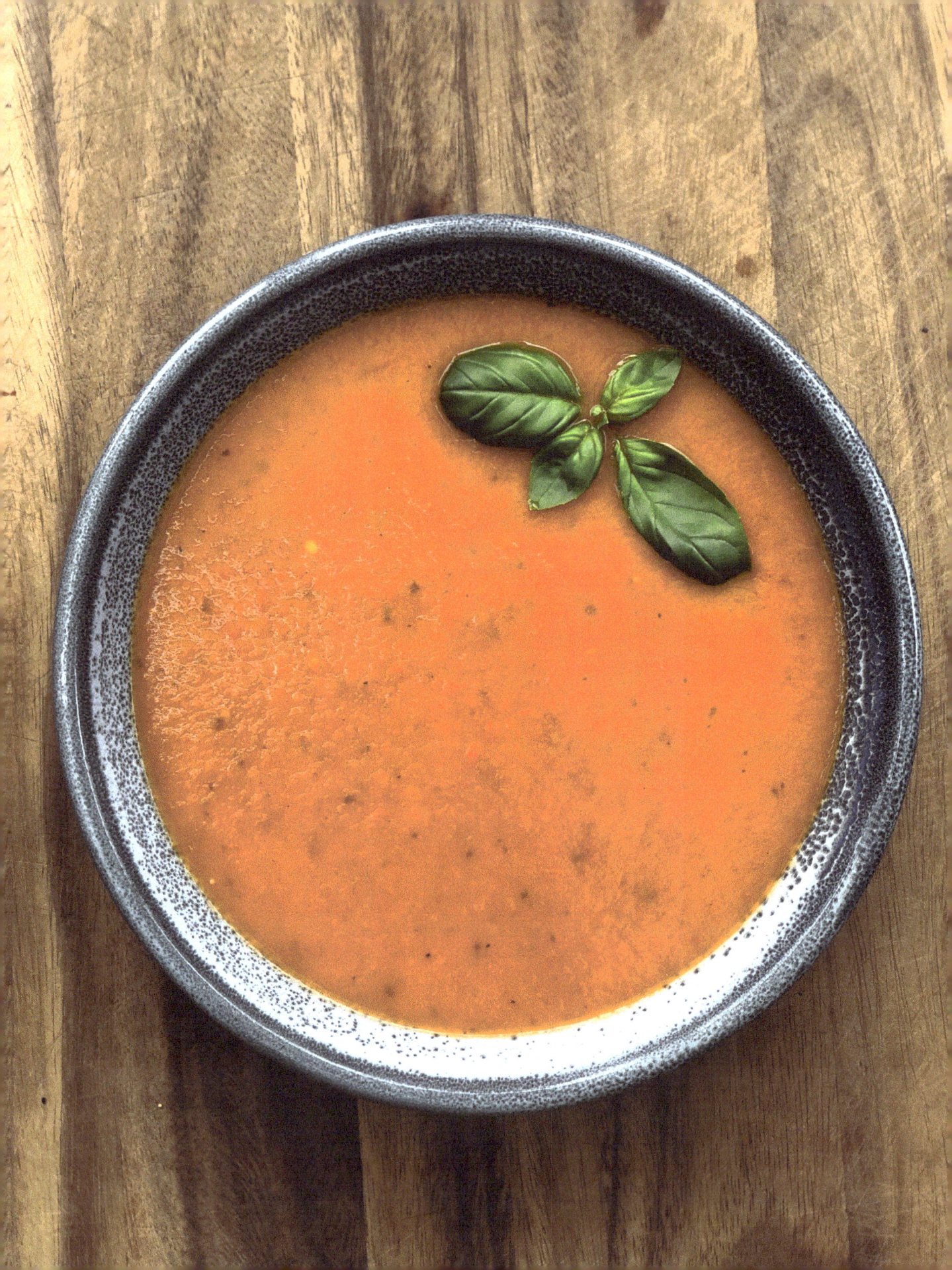

ROASTED TOMATO AND BASIL SOUP

PREPARATION TIME
10 MINUTES

COOKING TIME
50 MINUTES

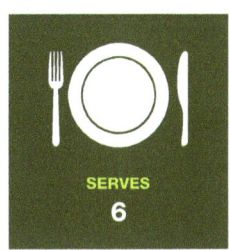
SERVES
6

INGREDIENTS:

1.8kg mixed tomatoes – common tomatoes mixed with 2 punnets cherry tomatoes work well. If you can find slightly overripe seconds, these work best!
45ml garlic infused olive oil
Salt and freshly ground black pepper
1 red capsicum, deseeded and diced
3 medium potatoes, diced
40gm tomato paste
1 litre low FODMAP vegetable broth
35gm lightly packed fresh basil leaves, roughly torn. Reserve some for garnish.

METHOD:

1. Preheat oven to 220°C.
2. Wash and cut tomatoes in halves.
3. Place tomatoes on a baking tray, drizzle with 30ml garlic infused oil. Sprinkle with salt and pepper and roast for 25 minutes until soft and charred on the tops.
4. Heat 15ml of oil in a medium-sized saucepan over medium-high heat. Add capsicum and potato.
5. Cook while occasionally stirring until the potato begins to crisp approximately 6–7 minutes.
6. Add the tomato paste, mixing through the potato and capsicum.
7. Pour in the stock, season to taste.
8. Cover saucepan and bring to a boil.
9. Reduce heat to low, simmering for 15 minutes or until potato is tender. Add the tomatoes and basil to the broth continue to simmer until the basil is just soft approximately 2 minutes.
10. Blend soup until smooth.
11. Sprinkle with extra basil.

For a smoother soup, you may strain it to remove excess tomato skins. I like the skins as it creates a more rustic texture and increases the fibre content.

ROOT VEGETABLE SOUP

This is such a winter warming soup. So hearty and filling, you finish your bowl with a great big smile of contentment.

PREPARATION TIME: 40 MINUTES
COOKING TIME: 2 HOURS
SERVES: 6

INGREDIENTS:

30ml garlic infused olive oil
2 medium carrots
2 large potatoes
1 turnip
1 swede
1 parsnip
1 stalk celery
150gm diced JAP or Kent Pumpkin
125gm chana dal – thoroughly washed and rinsed
5gm GF vegemite or alternative
Himalayan sea salt and Black pepper to taste
Water

METHOD:

1. Slice celery quite thin.
2. Dice the carrots, potatoes, turnip, swede, parsnip and pumpkin.
3. Heat oil in a large saucepan and add celery.
4. Fry until starts to go soft.
5. Add the diced vegetables and mix and coat in the oil.
6. Pour in enough water to cover the vegies.
7. Add chana dal.
8. Bring to the boil, once boiled add vegemite and salt to taste.
9. Simmer for 2 hours.

Extra water may need to be added during the simmer phase. Adjust seasoning accordingly.
Exceeding ½ cup cooked chana dahl may cause discomfort, therefore keep servings to a tolerable level.

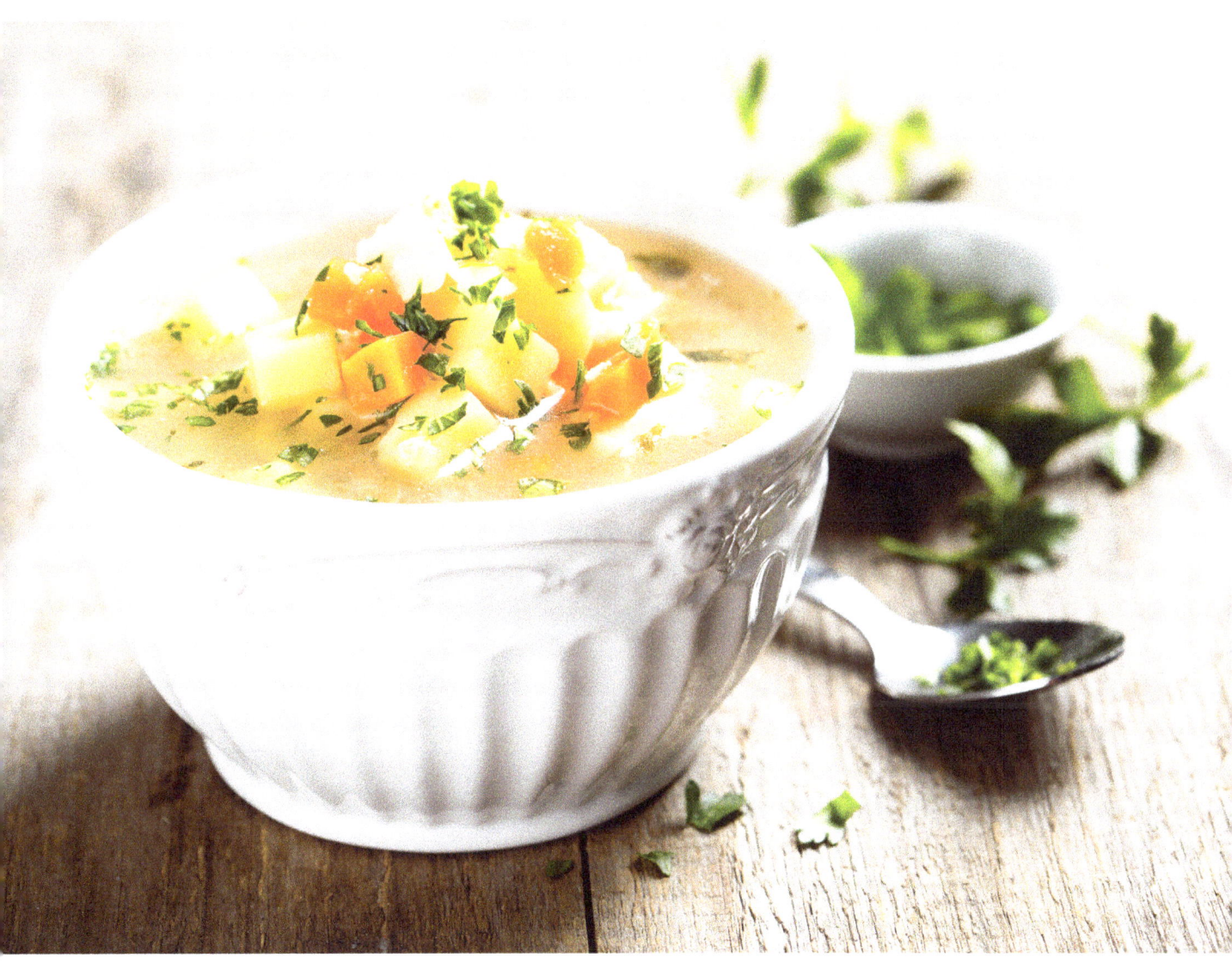

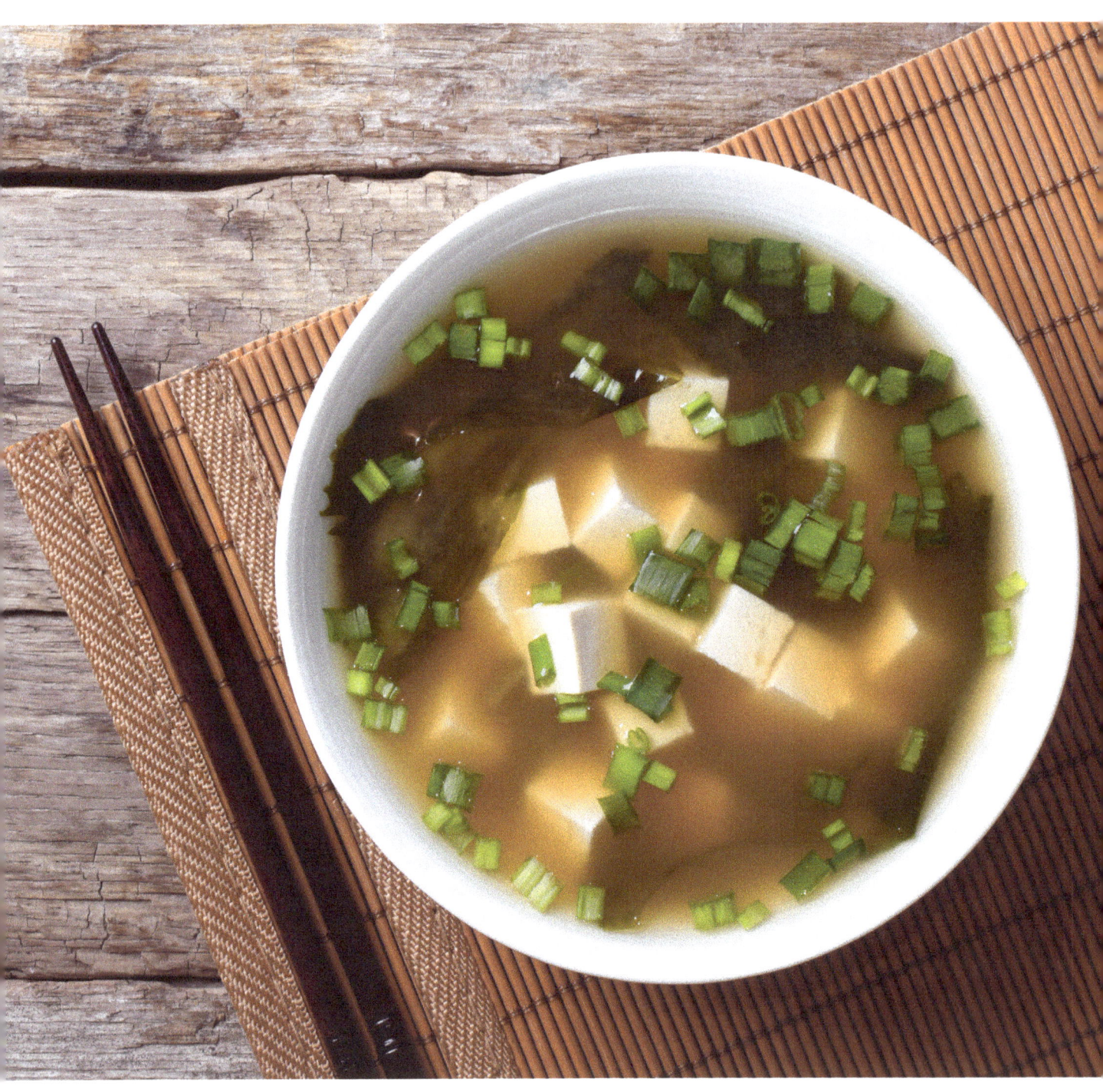

MISO EASY SOUP

I love this simple soup. I often have it when running out the door in the morning or a simple morning or afternoon pick me up. The salty richness provides a satisfaction and I feel warm and happy after I drink it.

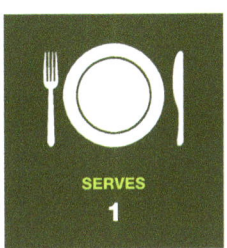

INGREDIENTS:

200ml water
8gm GF miso paste (I prefer Genmai)
2gm wakame flakes
30gm soft tofu – diced small
Spring onions, sliced, green tops only (optional)

METHOD:

1. Bring water to boil, then let sit for 5 minutes to just go off the boil.
2. Place miso paste, tofu and wakame flakes in mug.
3. Pour water into mug and wait for wakame to soften.
4. Drink and enjoy.

NB: Please note, not all miso is gluten free. Ensure you choose a rice miso. Genmai is my personal favourite.

If you like a stronger more robust flavour, add more miso.

MINESTRONE

PREPARATION TIME
30 MINUTES

COOKING TIME
1 HOUR 20 MINUTES

SERVES
4

INGREDIENTS:

30gm garlic infused oil
2 sticks celery
2 medium carrots
2 medium potatoes
140gm shredded green cabbage
½ small zucchini
440gm can fire roasted tomatoes
50gm tomato paste
1x 400gm can chickpeas, drained and rinsed
110gm GF risoni or other small pasta
10ml liquid smoke (optional)
1ltr FODMAP friendly vegetable stock
Himalayan sea salt and pepper to taste
Basil leaves for decoration

METHOD:

1. Dice potatoes, carrots and celery.

2. Heat oil in a large saucepan.

3. Add celery, potatoes, carrots and fry for 5 minutes.

4. Dice and add zucchini.

5. When slightly cooked, add stock, tomatoes, tomato paste, green cabbage, liquid smoke and chickpeas.

6. Bring to the boil, simmer for 30 minutes.

7. Add pasta and simmer for a further 30 minutes, stirring occasionally.

8. Add salt and pepper to taste.

9. Top with some basil leaves.

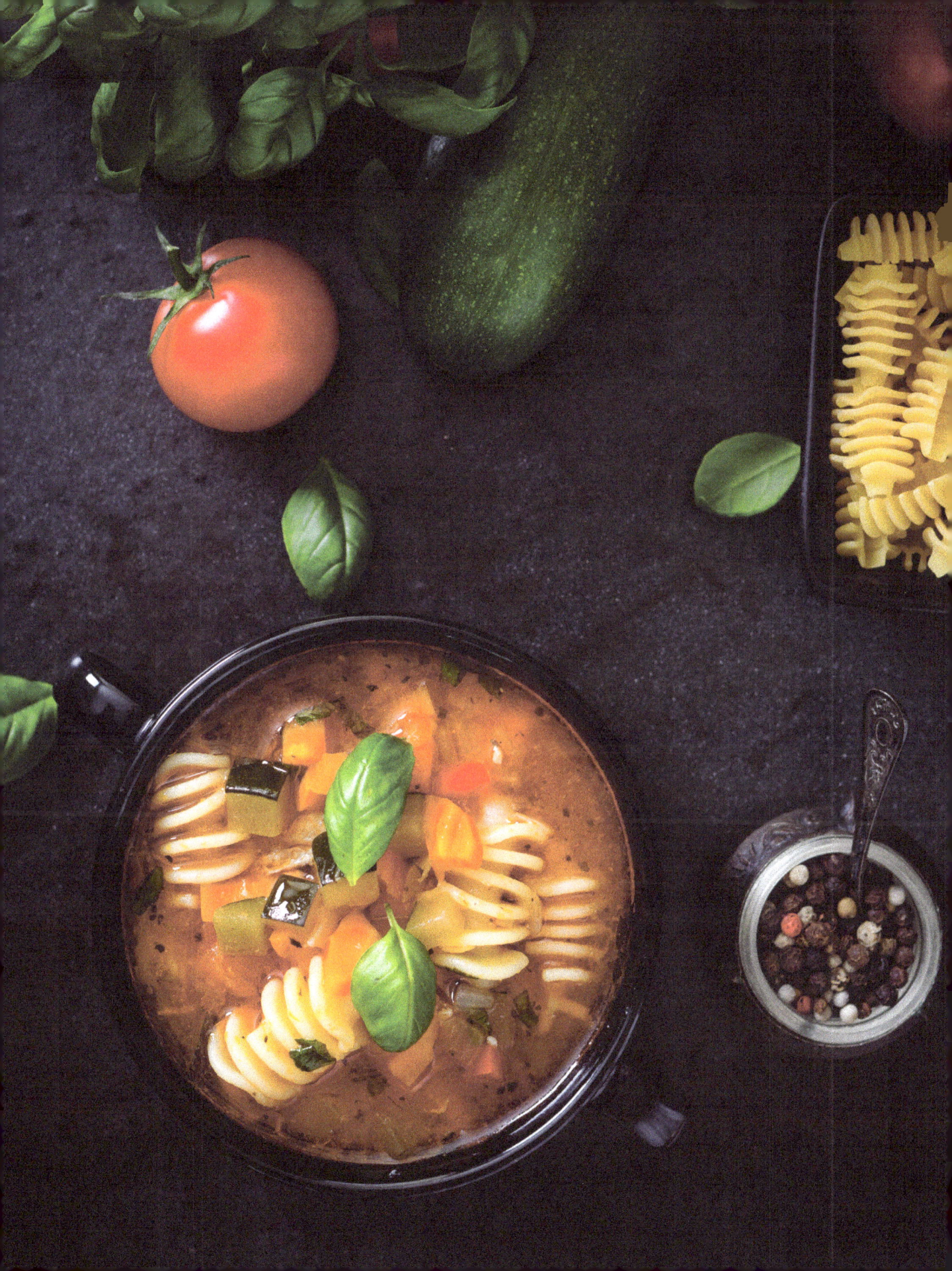

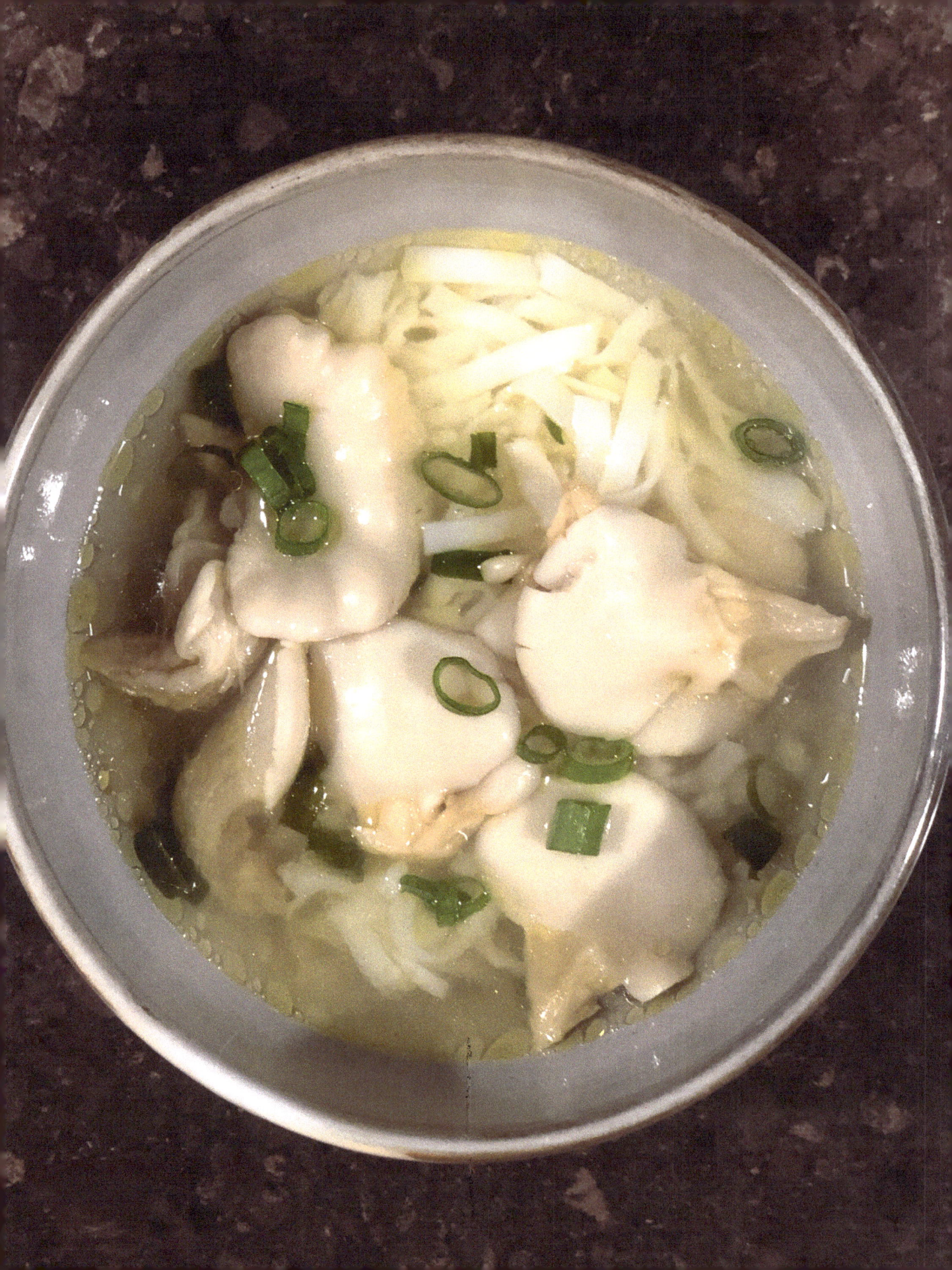

OYSTER MUSHROOM BROTH

Anyone who knows me, knows just how much I love medicinal mushrooms and how they are a regular in our house. I always have them on hand whether they are fresh or in a powdered form to add to hot drinks or dishes. Lucky for me oyster mushrooms are allowed in the low **FODMAP** diet, so this is one I get to enjoy with the family. This is such an easy recipe that is rich in antioxidants, supports cancer cell destruction, heart healthy and aids in reducing cholesterol. What more can you ask for?

This simple recipe is rich in flavour and continues to make the mushrooms the hero of the dish.

PREPARATION TIME 20 MINUTES
COOKING TIME 10 MINUTES
SERVES 4

INGREDIENTS:

30ml garlic infused oil
600gm oyster mushrooms
2 litres low Fodmap vegetable stock
3 spring onions, green parts only
5gm parsley
Salt and pepper to taste

METHOD:

1. Wash oyster mushrooms and cut into mouthful size pieces.
2. Thinly slice spring onions, reserving a small handful for garnish.
3. Heat oil in a saucepan, once hot, add mushrooms and spring onions and cook for 2 minutes.
4. Add liquid stock and bring to the boil.
5. Add salt and pepper to taste.
6. Divide into bowls, garnishing with parsley and reserved spring onions.

VIETNAMESE PHO

This is a bit more involved to cook but definitely worth the wait.
I love the way the flavours all combine to create a melody on the palate.

PREPARATION TIME
40 MINUTES

COOKING TIME
1 HOUR 15 MINUTES

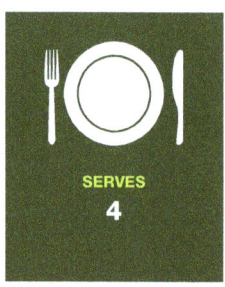
SERVES
4

INGREDIENTS:

SOUP

2 cinnamon sticks
2 cloves
1 star anise
2gm coriander seeds
6gm black peppercorns
1 leek, green part only, washed thoroughly and thinly sliced
4cm piece fresh ginger, grated
1 litre vegetable broth
30ml GF soy sauce
200gm vermicelli rice noodle
10gm coconut sugar
10ml vegan fish sauce (optional)
Salt and pepper to taste

TOFU

250gm firm tofu – cut into 1.5cm cubes
30gm cornflour
5gm coriander powder
Salt and pepper to taste
Garlic infused oil

TOPPINGS

Fresh basil leaves
Fresh coriander
Fresh mint
Red chilli – Sliced
Spring onions – green parts only, sliced
Lime
Oyster mushrooms – lightly fried
Bean sprouts

For an extra buzz, you can leave the leeks in the soup as I do but it does take away from traditional pho.

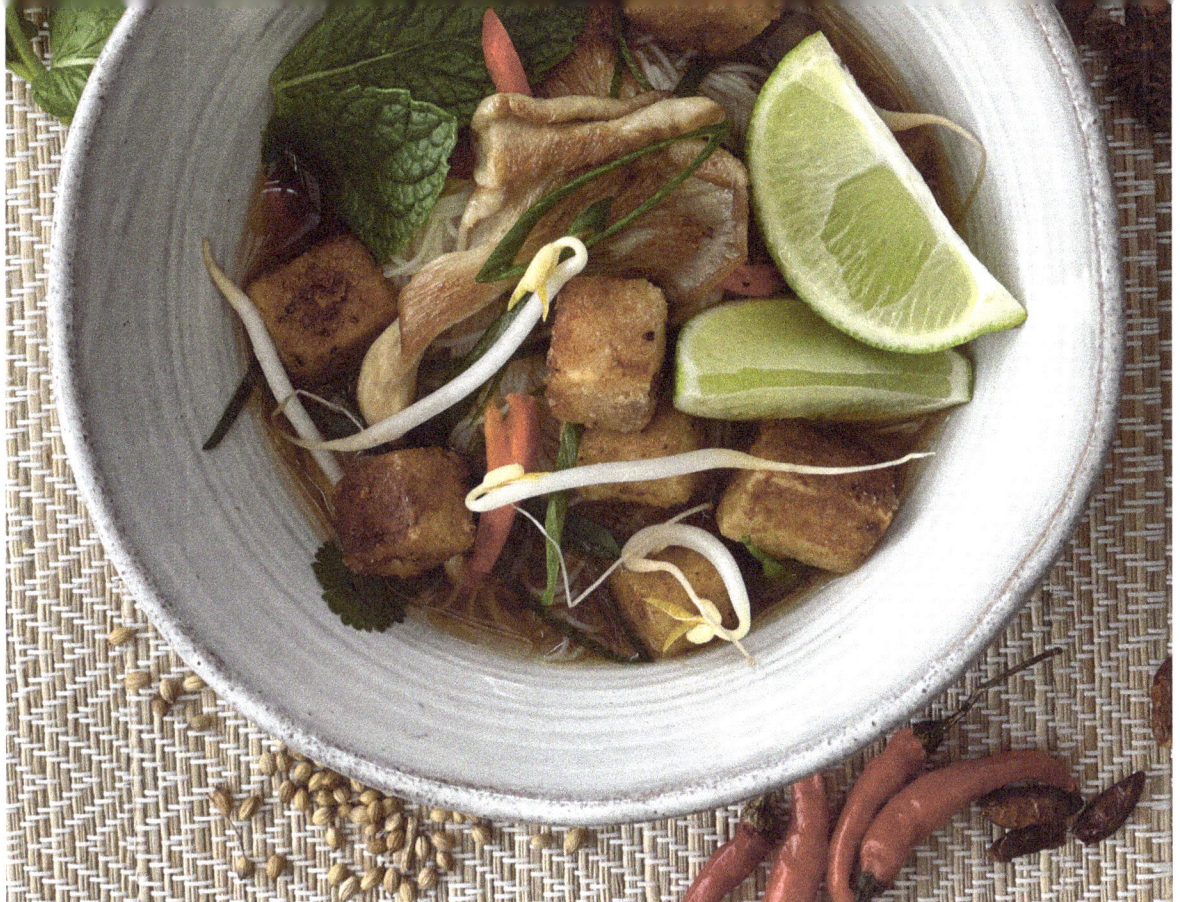

METHOD:

1. Drain tofu, wrap in a towel and squeeze excess moisture out. Set aside.
2. Boil kettle. Place vermicelli rice noodles in a bowl, pour boiling water over them, set aside.
3. In a large saucepan, over moderate heat, add cinnamon sticks, cloves, star anise, coriander seeds and peppercorns.
4. Cook for 3 minutes until fragrant.
5. Add grated ginger, leeks, vegetable broth and tamari. Season to taste.
6. Bring to the boil. Once boiled, reduce heat, place lid on saucepan and simmer approximately 40 minutes.
7. Combine corn-starch, salt, pepper and coriander powder in a medium size bowl. Add tofu, a few at a time, thoroughly coating each piece as you go.
8. Place oil in a large fry pan and heat pan to a high heat. Add tofu cooking each side until they are brown and crispy.
9. Add an extra splash of tamari to the pan, quickly tossing tofu until they are all coated with the soy sauce. This will spit so if you have a lid, place it over tofu as soon as you add the tamari. Remove from heat and set aside.
10. Once broth has completed simmering, add sugar, vegan fish sauce (optional) and salt and pepper to taste.
11. Once combined, strain soup through muslin cloth. Further season to taste with salt, pepper and tamari.
12. Drain noodles and divide into 4 bowls.
13. Ladle broth equally into each bowl.
14. Top with tofu and chosen toppings.
15. Serve immediately and enjoy.

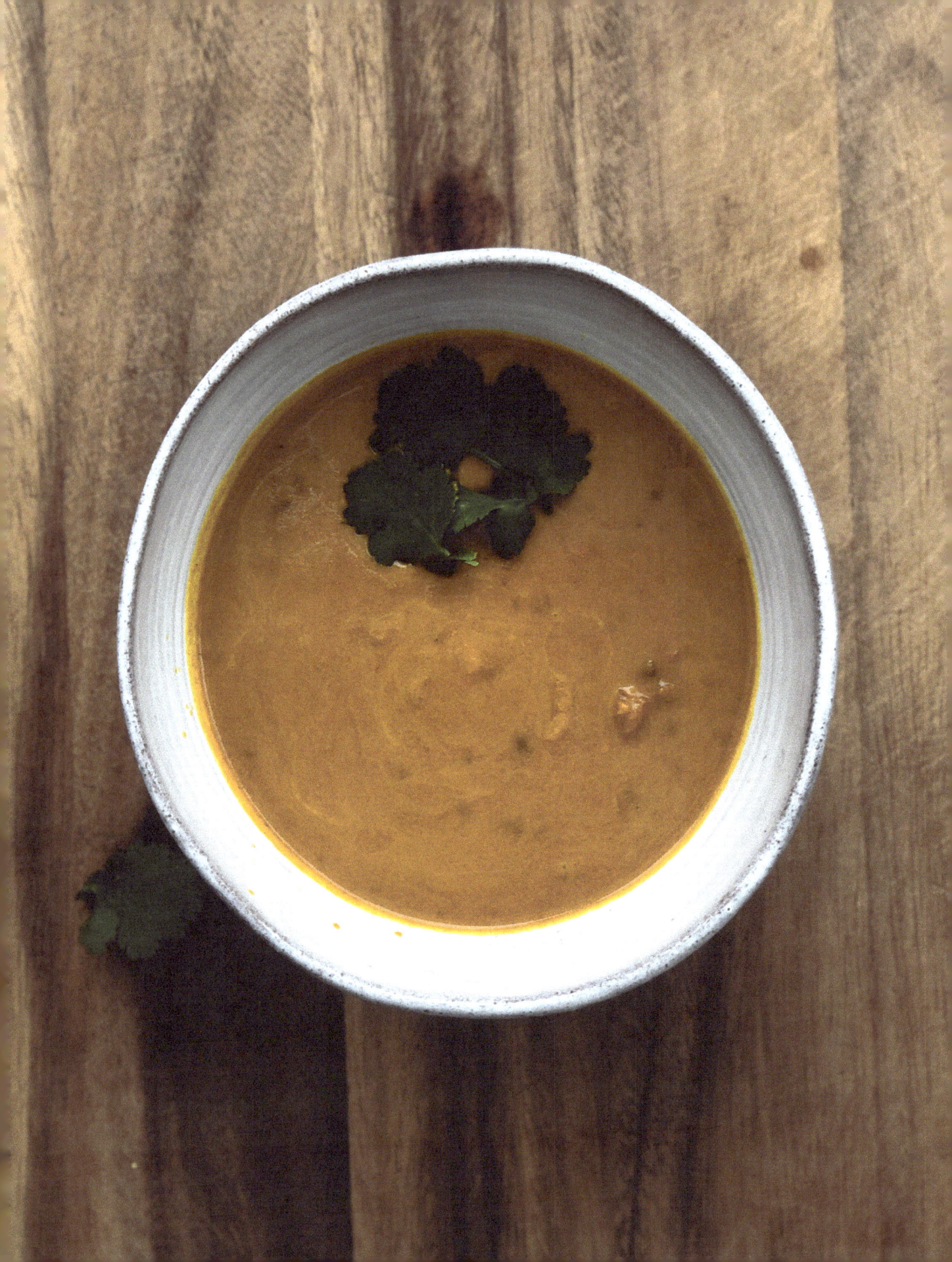

CREAMY LENTIL SOUP

Very much a comfort food, this thick creamy soup is a must on a cold winter's night. Full of vitamins and minerals and rich in fibre, it is a quick and easy Saturday night fix.

PREPARATION TIME
15 MINUTES

COOKING TIME
20 MINUTES

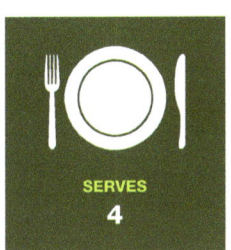
SERVES
4

INGREDIENTS:

1x 400gm can brown lentils
1x 400gm can diced tomatoes
1x 400gm can coconut cream
125ml water
20ml garlic infused oil
10gm ground cumin
10gm fresh ginger, grated
5gm fresh oregano, finely chopped.
5gm paprika
2.5gm chilli flakes
2gm cinnamon
2gm turmeric
Salt and pepper to taste
Coriander
Vegan sour cream (optional)

METHOD:

1. Drain lentils and rinse.
2. Place everything except fresh coriander, salt and pepper in a non-stick saucepan.
3. Bring to a preboil over a medium heat, to prevent sticking.
4. Reduce heat and ensure a constant simmer for 20 minutes.
5. Season to taste with salt and pepper.
6. Divide between 4 bowls and garnish with fresh coriander.
7. For an added touch, try a dollop of sour cream.

60ml is the recommended dose of coconut cream so if you are particularly sensitive, don't serve a large bowl.

COCONUT AND SWEET POTATO SOUP

PREPARATION TIME
20 MINUTES

COOKING TIME
18 MINUTES

SERVES
4

INGREDIENTS:

15gm coconut oil
15gm garlic infused olive oil
450gm sweet potato
1 stick celery finely diced
5gm grated ginger
15gm low FODMAP medium-hot curry paste
600ml low FODMAP vegetable stock
200ml coconut cream
Juice of 1 lime
2gm dried chilli
175gm baby spinach (optional)
Himalayan salt and pepper to taste
Vegan sour cream
Chilli flakes

METHOD:

1. Peel and cut potato into 1 cm cubes.
2. In a large saucepan, heat oils and add potato, celery, ginger and curry paste.
3. Fry for 5 minutes or until golden brown.
4. Add stock, coconut cream, lime juice and chilli.
5. Bring to the boil, cover and simmer until potatoes are tender. Approx. 15 minutes.
6. Roughly puree half of the soup leaving some chunky pieces.
7. If using spinach, add now and cook until leaves are wilted and soup is heated through.
8. Season to taste, garnish with sour cream and a sprinkle of chilli flakes.
9. Serve and ENJOY.

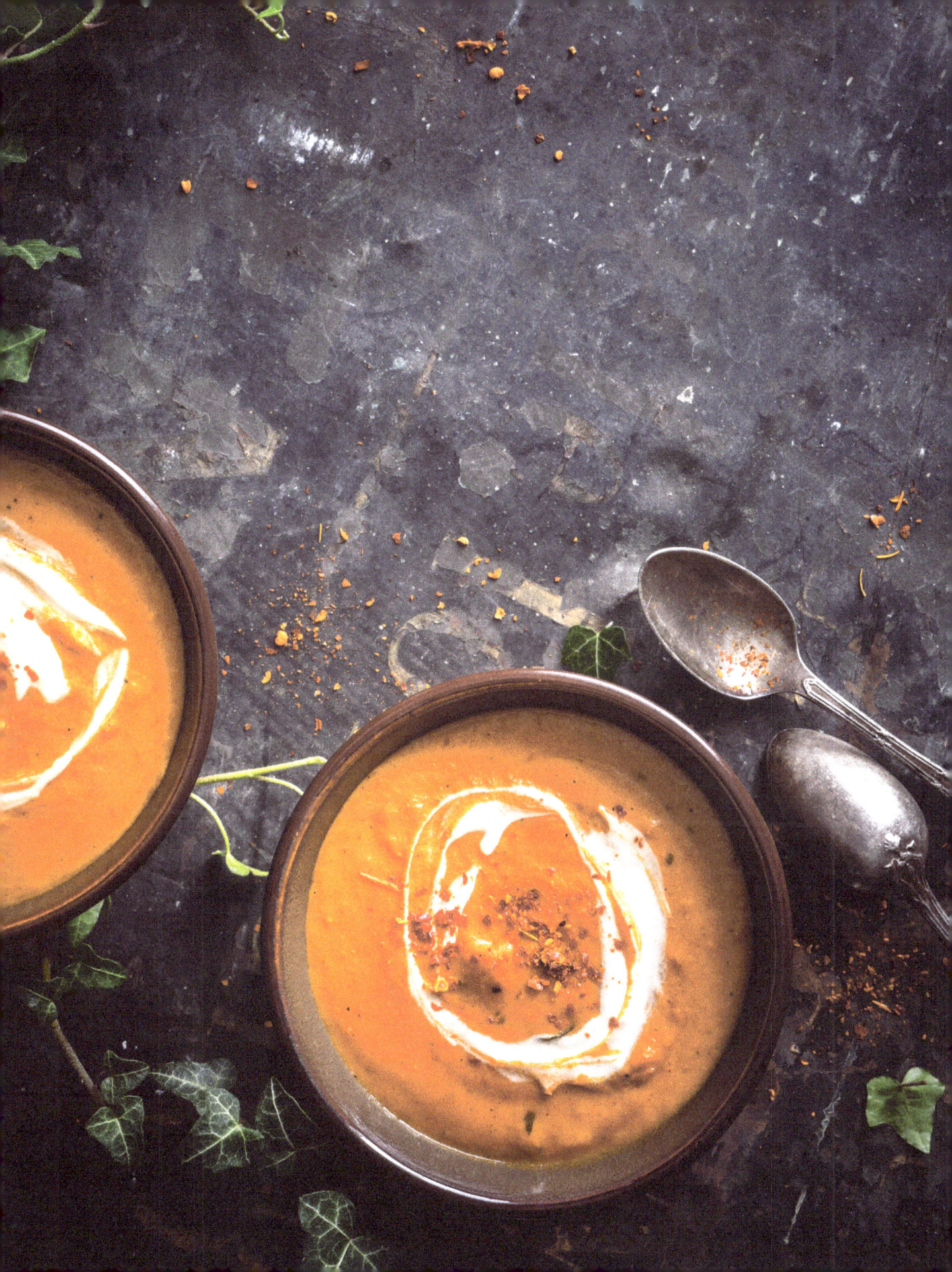

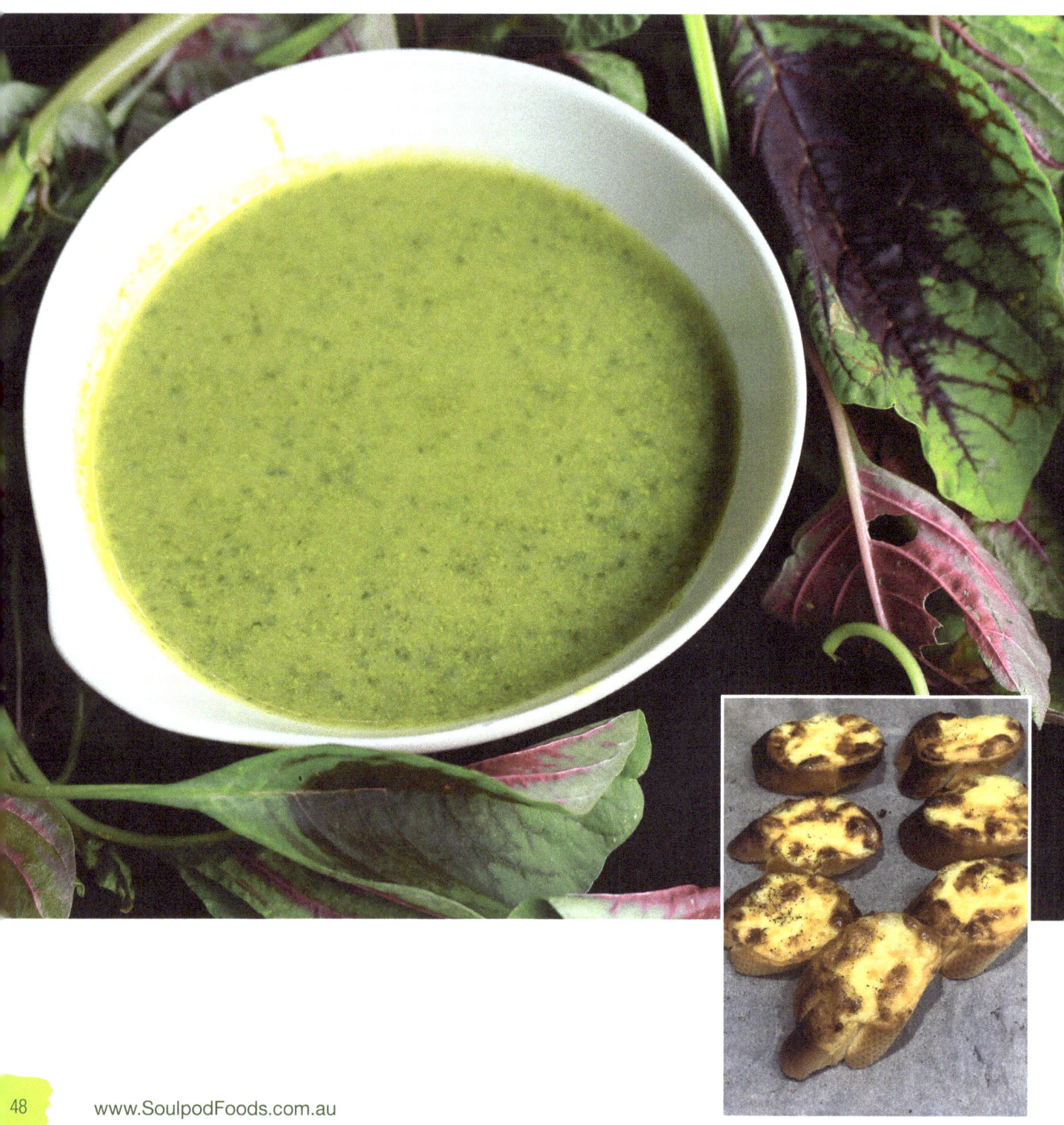

SPINACH SOUP
WITH CHEESY CROUTONS

PREPARATION TIME
10 MINUTES

COOKING TIME
20 MINUTES

SERVES
6

INGREDIENTS:

30ml garlic infused olive oil
20gm coconut oil
750gm potato
250gm spinach leaves
5gm nutmeg
1.5 litres low FODMAP vegetable stock
60gm vegan sour cream
100gm plant-based shredded tasty cheese
GF baguette, cut into 1 cm slices
Salt and Pepper to taste
Extra vegan sour cream

METHOD:

1. Heat olive oil and the coconut oil in a large saucepan.
2. Add the potatoes and fry for 2 minutes, add spinach and nutmeg, cooking for a further few minutes until spinach is starting to wilt.
3. Add stock, season to taste and bring to the boil.
4. Once boiling, reduce heat, cover and simmer 15 minutes or until potatoes are tender. Set aside.
5. After soup has cooled a little, using a hand blender, blend until smooth. Season to taste, set aside.
6. Mix cheese with the sour cream.
7. Toast the slices of baguette, then spread the cheese mix on one side.
8. Season with black pepper. Place under grill and cook until golden.
9. Dish up the soup into bowls and enjoy with the cheese croutons.

For a creamier soup add a spoon of sour cream and mix through.

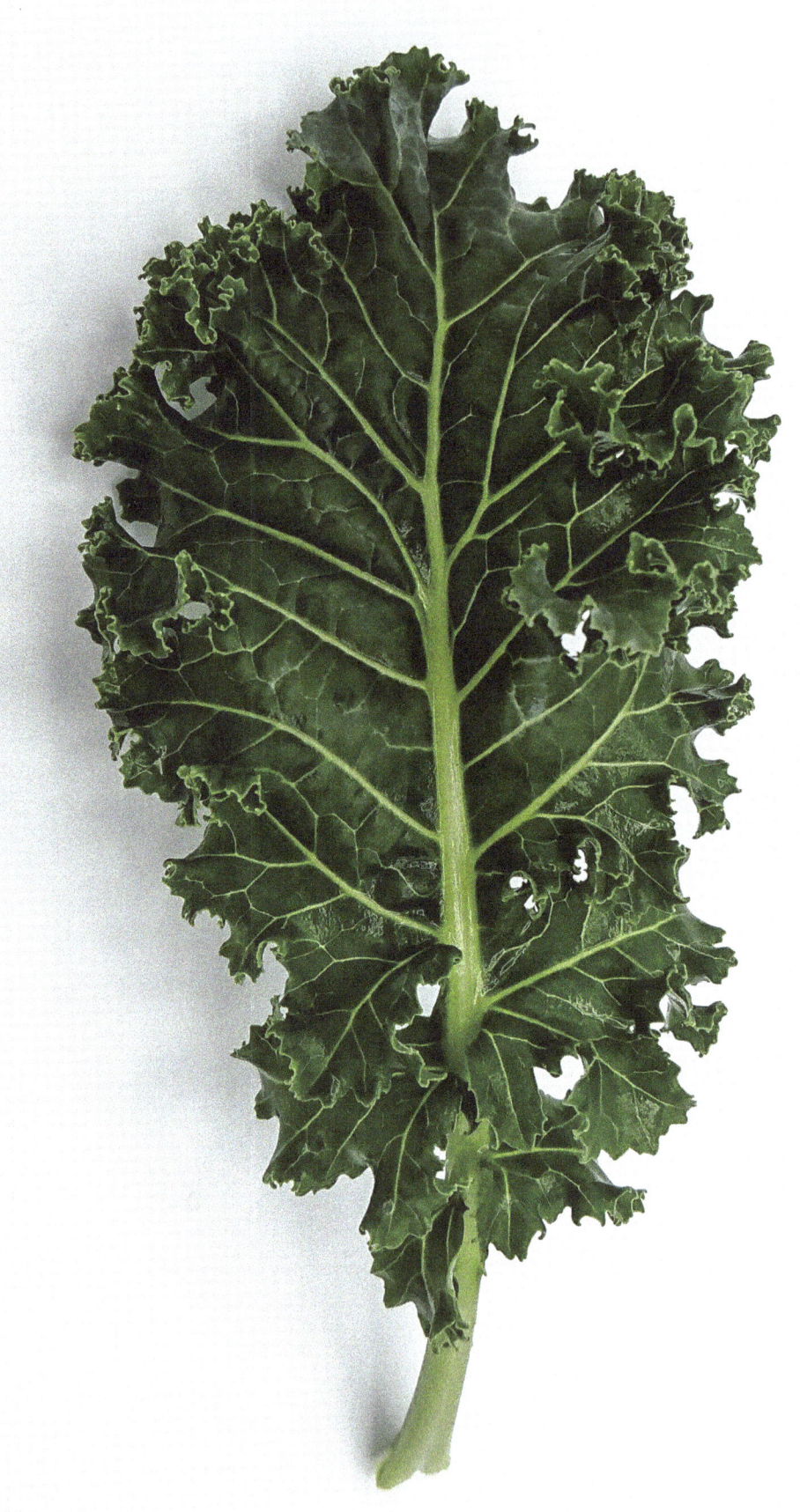

CHAPTER 3
Salads

In a world where you can be anything,
BE KIND.

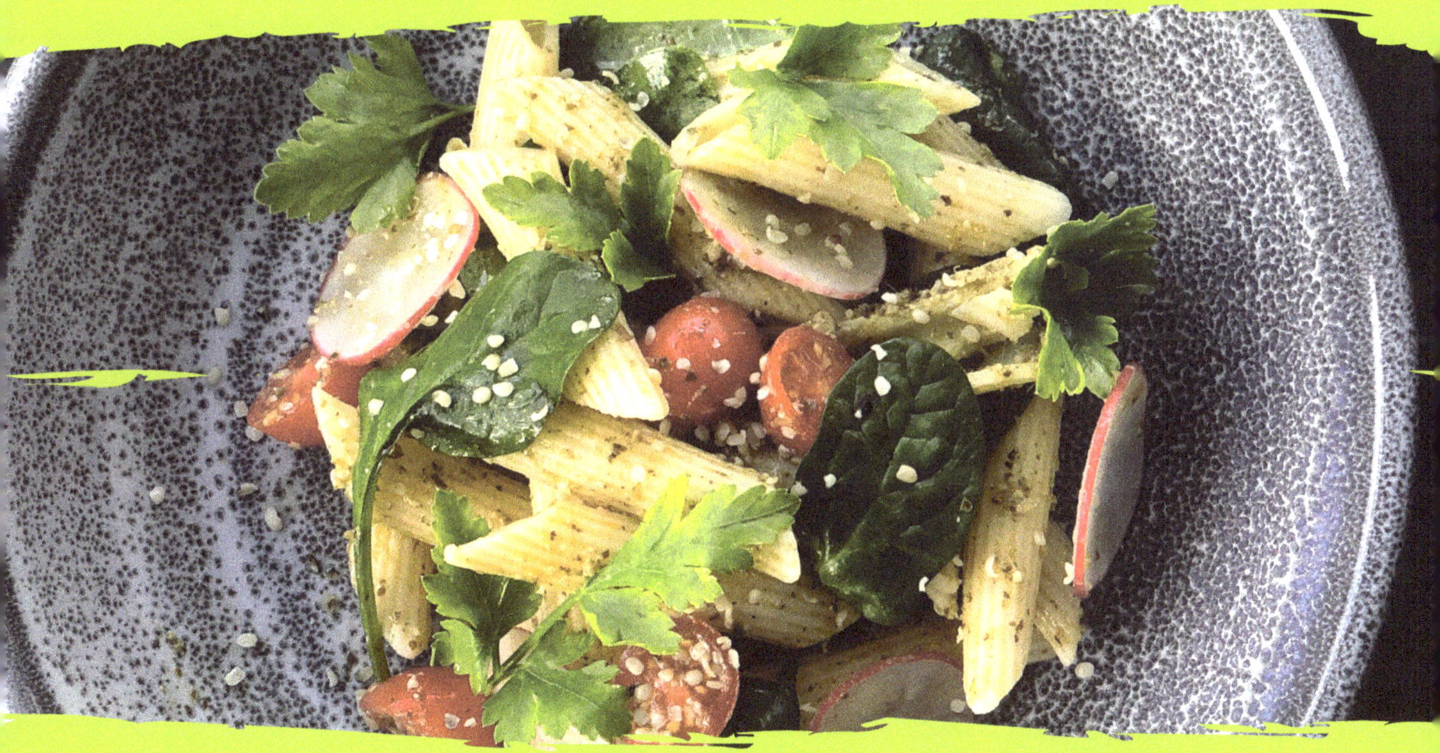

I love salads. We are so lucky to live in Australia with our vast variety of available fresh produce. Fruit and vegetables are rich in enzymes that assist us in breaking down our foods and digest them. They are also rich in anti-inflammatory, antioxidant, antiparasitic, antiviral and antibacterial properties. Why wouldn't we include salads in our diet daily??

WARM SUMMER HEMP PASTA SALAD

PREPARATION TIME
15 MINUTES

COOKING TIME
10 MINUTES

SERVES
6

INGREDIENTS:

100gm GF pasta
15ml hemp oil
1 punnet cherry tomatoes
4 chopped radishes
10gm hemp seeds
Lots of baby spinach
1 quantity macadamia nut pesto

METHOD:

1. Cook pasta according to directions.
2. Drain and place back in saucepan.
3. Add pesto and oil stirring to completely coat the pasta.
4. Add chopped cherry tomatoes, chopped radish, hemp seeds and spinach. Mix through.
5. Season to taste. Serve immediately.

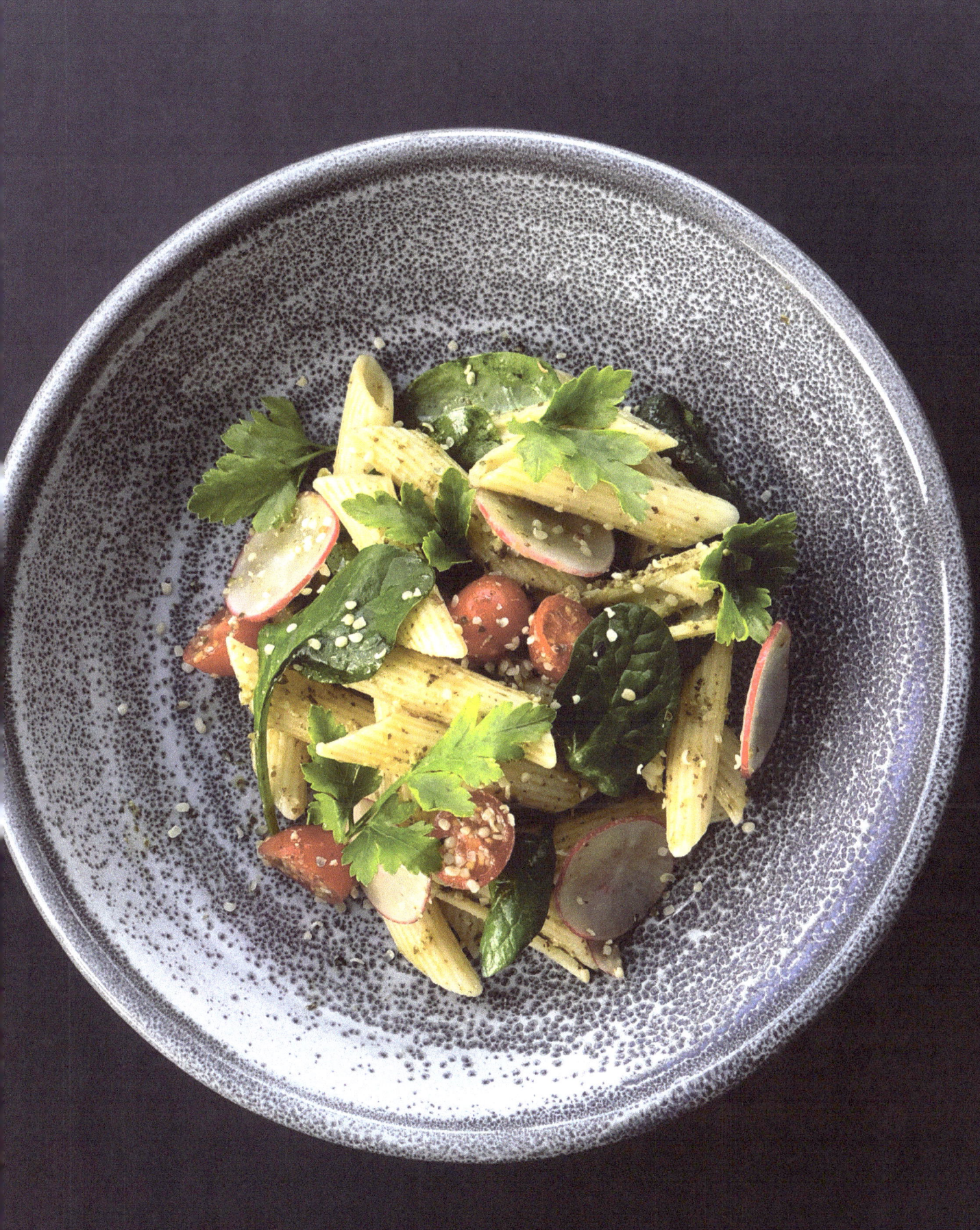

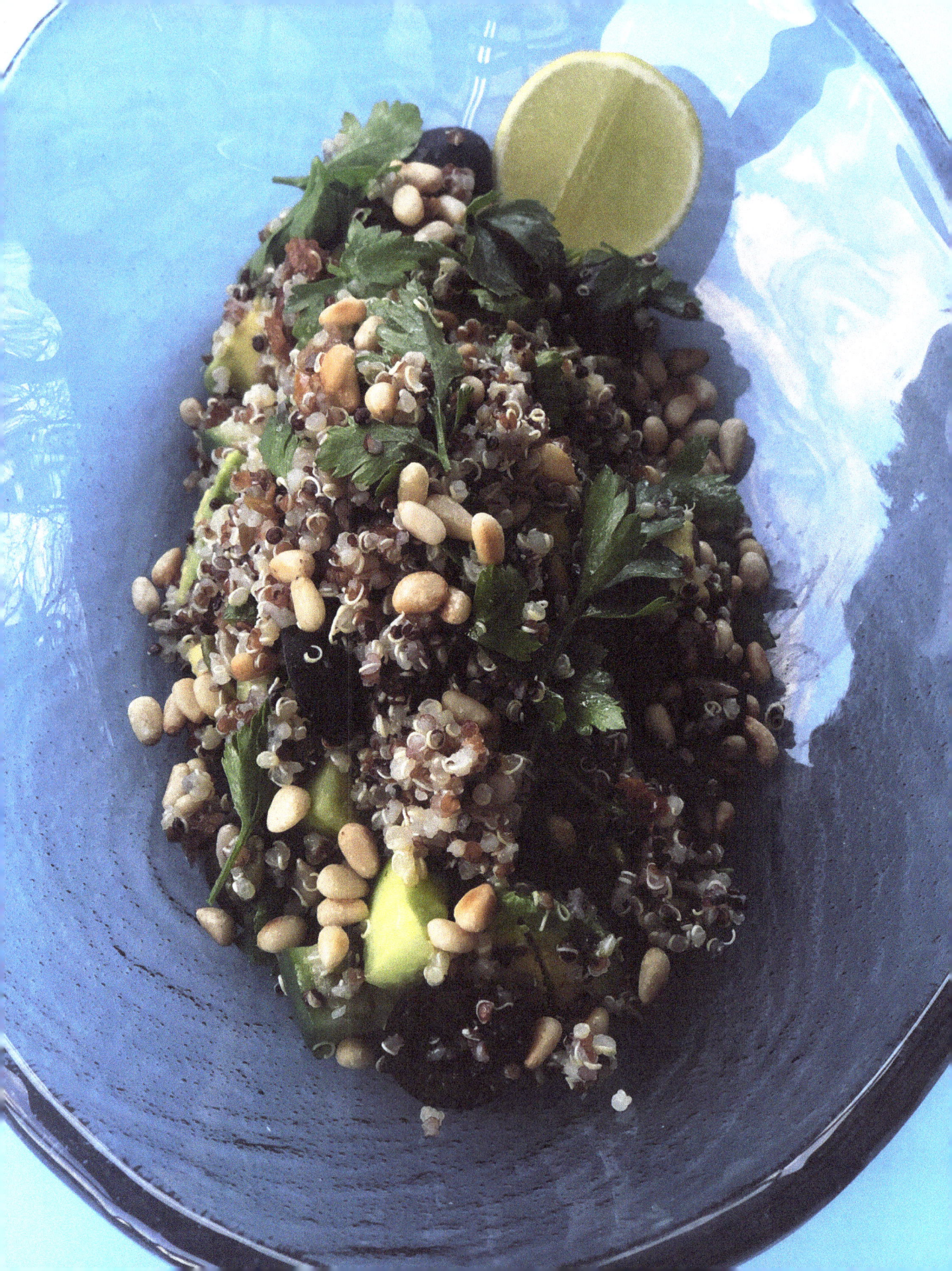

JEWEL QUINOA SALAD

PREPARATION TIME: 20 MINUTES
COOKING TIME: 15 MINUTES
SERVES: 8

INGREDIENTS:

180gm quinoa
500ml water
1 avocado – diced
5 semidried tomatoes- thinly sliced
1 Lebanese cucumber – diced with skin on
10 Olives halved
70gm toasted pinenuts
½ bunch flat leaf parsley – roughly chopped
30gm of pumpkin seeds (this adds a great crunch)
30gm sunflower kernels
Himalayan sea salt and pepper to taste
Squeeze lemon juice

METHOD:

1. Rinse quinoa thoroughly under running water until all the 'soapiness' disappears.
2. Place quinoa in saucepan with the water and bring to the boil.
3. Place lid on saucepan, turn heat down and simmer for 10 minutes.
4. Once cooked, leave the lid on and turn off the heat. Let the quinoa sit for 10 minutes to finish absorbing water.
5. Allow quinoa to cool.
6. Prepare all other ingredients ready for the salad.
7. Place cooled quinoa into a bowl and add prepared ingredients.
8. Pour over the dressing.

You can eat this as a warm salad or wait until the quinoa completely cools down.

SMOKED PAPRIKA AND ROASTED PUMPKIN SALAD

PREPARATION TIME
15 MINUTES

COOKING TIME
20 MINUTES

SERVES
4

INGREDIENTS:

260gm pumpkin
1gm paprika
pinch Himalayan sea salt
30ml rice bran oil
6gm sesame seeds.
10gm almonds.
Handful of baby spinach
35gm pinenuts
50gm macadamia feta

METHOD:

1. Preheat oven 200°C.

2. Peel, cube and coat pumpkin in ricebran oil. Sprinkle with paprika and salt and bake until cooked.

3. Lightly toast sesame seeds, pinenuts and almonds in a dry fry pan. Remove from pan and let sit on paper towel to cool.

4. Once cool, roughly chop the almonds.

5. Once pumpkin has baked and cooled, place in a bowl with almonds, sesame seeds, pinenuts and baby spinach.

6. Sprinkle with macadamias feta, serve and enjoy.

www.SoulpodFoods.com.au

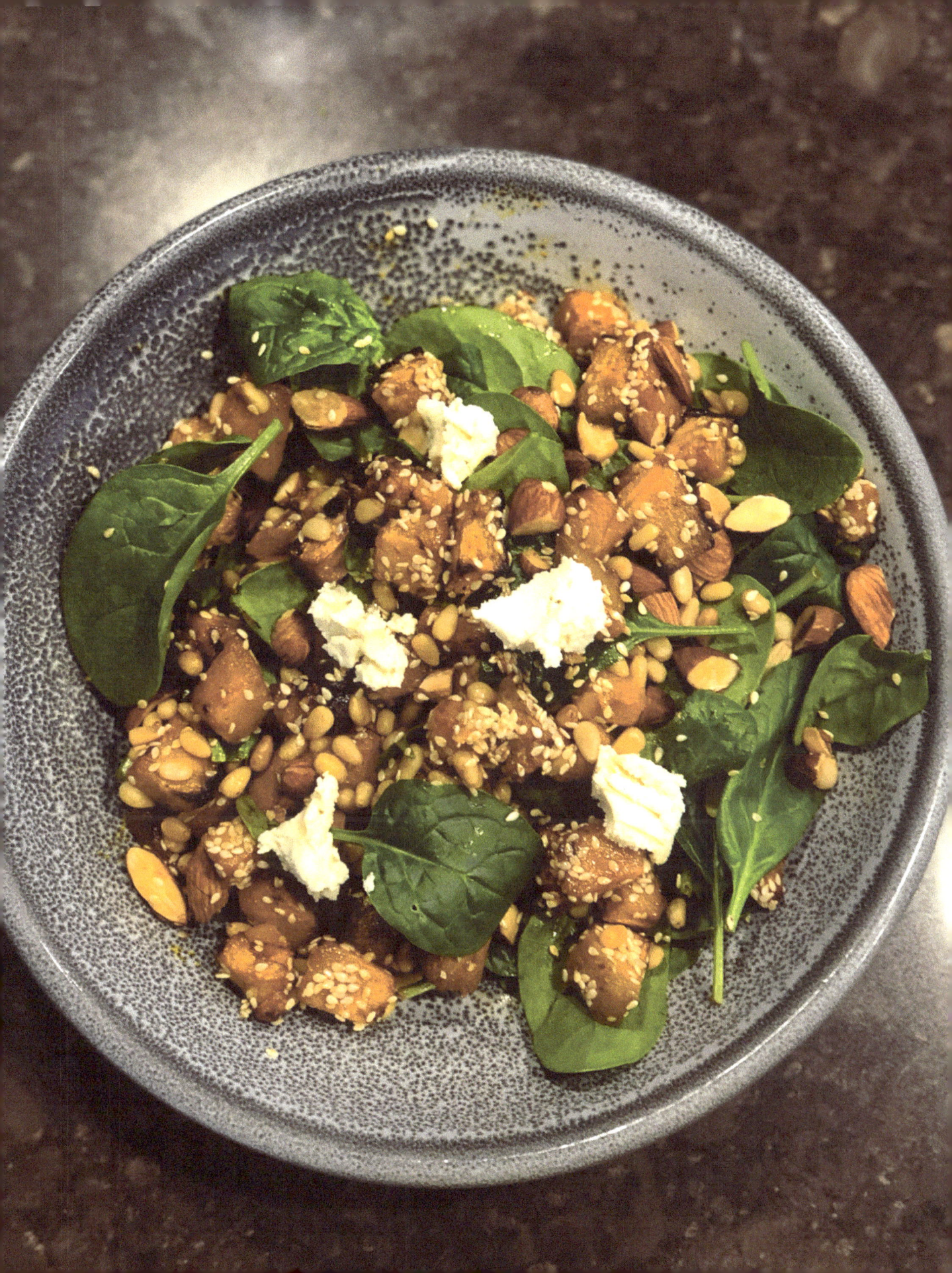

OLD SCHOOL TROPICAL SALAD

PREPARATION TIME 15 MINUTES

SERVES 6

INGREDIENTS:

400gm tin pineapple chunks
½ green pepper
½ red pepper
4 sticks celery
30gm roughly chopped walnuts
60gm vegan mayonnaise
lemon juice – as required

METHOD:

1. Dice peppers and celery, place in a bowl.
2. Drain pineapple, add to bowl.
3. Combine remaining ingredients and serve.

BABA GANOUSH

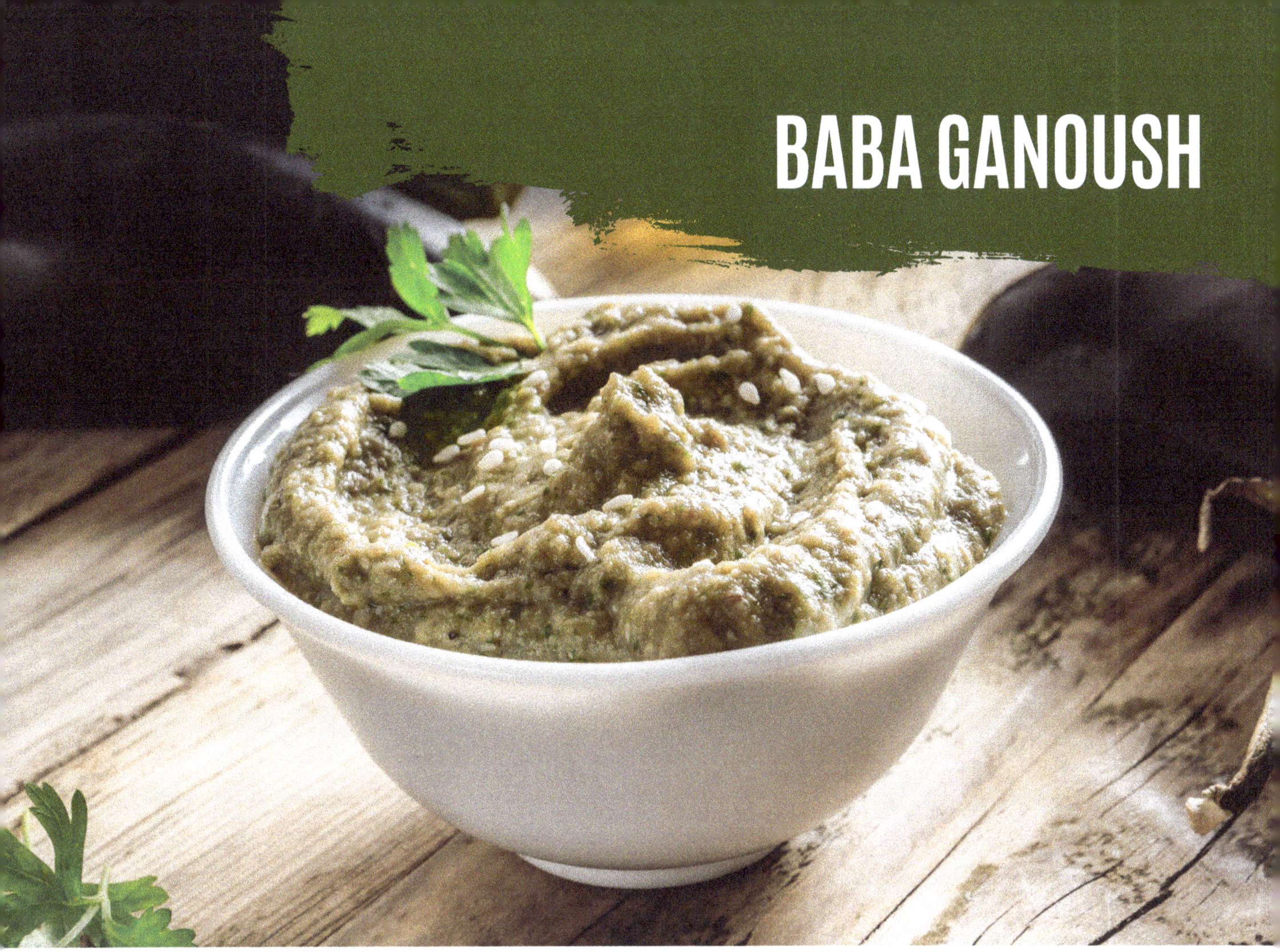

I adore this salad. This can be used as a side on the meal plate or used as a dip with crudites. I have used it in a wrap using marinated Mediterranean vegetables. It is so versatile and really packs a punch with flavour. One of my all-time favourites.

PREPARATION TIME
20 MINUTES

COOKING TIME
1 HOUR

SERVES
6

INGREDIENTS:

2 large eggplants
1 large lemon
10gm Himalayan sea salt
30ml garlic infused olive oil
½ stick celery – very finely chopped
4 sprigs parsley

METHOD:

1. Preheat oven to 180°C.
2. Bake eggplants 1 hour on a lined tray.
3. Let cool, scoop out insides into a bowl and mash with a fork.
4. Juice the lemon and add to eggplant.
5. Add remaining ingredients, blend thoroughly.
6. Refrigerate at least 6 hours before serving.

Blend longer for a smoother consistency.

Jodie Martin | **Chapter 3** Salads

NO-EGG SALAD

**PREPARATION TIME
10 MINUTES**

INGREDIENTS:

500gm block medium-firm tofu, drained and patted dry
70gm vegan mayonnaise – you can add up to 20gm more for a creamier texture
1 small celery stick finely diced
1.5gm turmeric
20gm nutritional yeast
10gm GF Dijon mustard
3 spring onions, green parts only, finely chopped
3gm kala namak
1gm turmeric
Chives, finely diced (optional)
salt and pepper to taste
1 pickle, finely diced (optional)

METHOD:

1. Chop tofu into small cubes.
2. Place tofu in a bowl and slightly mash.
3. Add remaining ingredients. Stir gently.
4. Add salt and pepper to taste.
5. This amount makes enough for four sandwiches with leafy greens. Double recipe if wanting it as a bowl of salad.

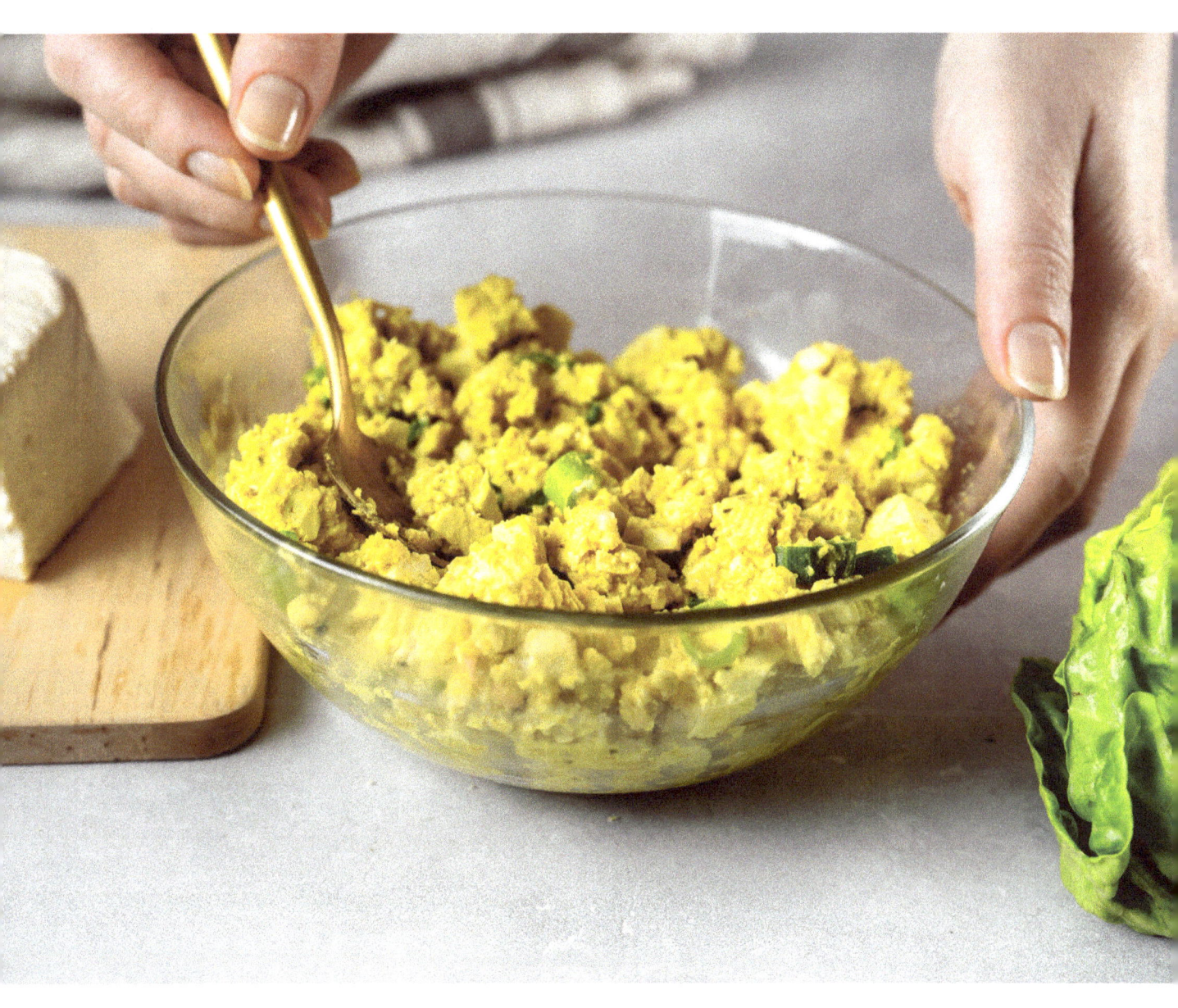

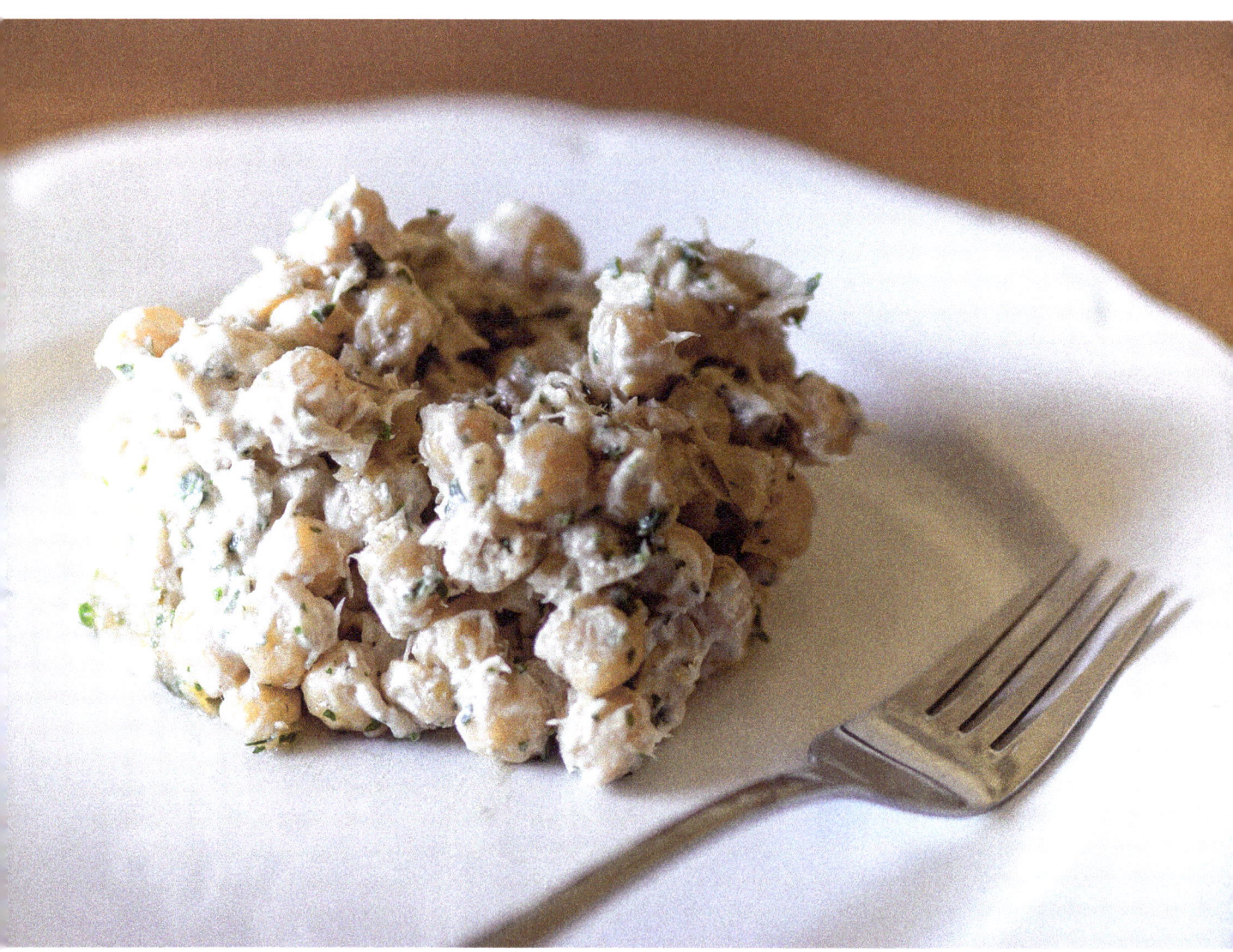

CHICKPEA TUNA SALAD

PREPARATION TIME
20 MINUTES

SERVES
4

INGREDIENTS:

400g can chickpeas, drained
45gm vegan mayonnaise – add more if wanting a creamier consistency
1 nori sheet, finely chopped
½ stick celery, finely chopped
15ml lemon juice
10 capers, finely chopped
15gm savoury yeast flakes
15ml tamari (add to taste)
10gm GF Dijon mustard
2.5ml white vinegar (or more to taste)
Himalayan sea salt and black pepper to taste

METHOD:

1. Add the chickpeas to a mixing bowl and roughly mash them with a fork.
2. Add in vegan mayonnaise, finely chopped nori, finely chopped celery, lemon juice, finely chopped capers, nutritional yeast, tamari, Dijon mustard, white vinegar and salt and pepper.
3. Add salt and pepper to taste.
4. Mix altogether and ready to serve.

This goes great in sandwiches with lettuce and nori rolls.

¼ cup of canned chickpeas is the recommended quantity on a low FODMAP diet. So, while enjoying this delicious dish, please watch portion size.

PEANUT SOBA NOODLE SALAD

PREPARATION TIME
15 MINUTES

COOKING TIME
10 MINUTES

SERVES
3
AS A MAIN

INGREDIENTS:

200gm 100% buckwheat soba noodles
5ml sesame oil
150gm edamame beans
250gm broccoli – cut into bite size pieces
30gm crunchy peanut butter
30ml tamari
15ml rice vinegar
5ml garlic infused olive oil
15gm ginger, freshly grated
2 spring onions, green tops only, thinly sliced
½ bunch coriander
2 limes
30gm chopped peanuts

METHOD:

1. Bring a medium size saucepan with water and salt to the boil. Place noodles in the water and cook for 4 minutes or until soft. Stir to separate the noodles. Once cooked through, drain noodles and rinse under cold water to stop the cooking process. Toss in sesame oil. Set aside.

2. Bring another medium size saucepan of water to the boil, add a pinch of salt and the edamame.

3. Allow to cook for 2 minutes, then add the broccoli and boil a further 3 minutes.

4. We are aiming for the vegies to maintain their vibrant green colour but able to bite through.

5. Drain edamame and broccoli. Rinse under cold water. Set aside.

6. Place peanuts in a dry fry pan and fry until they just turn a slight golden brown.

7. Place the peanut butter, tamari, rice vinegar, garlic infused oil, ginger and juice from 1 lime with a splash of boiling water in a bowl and whisk until thoroughly blended.

8. Place the broccoli and edamame into the bowl with the noodles along with the spring onions, 2/3 of the coriander and the dressing. Toss well to combine.

9. Divide equally into 3 bowls.

10. Over the top, scatter with chopped peanuts, remaining coriander and lime wedges.

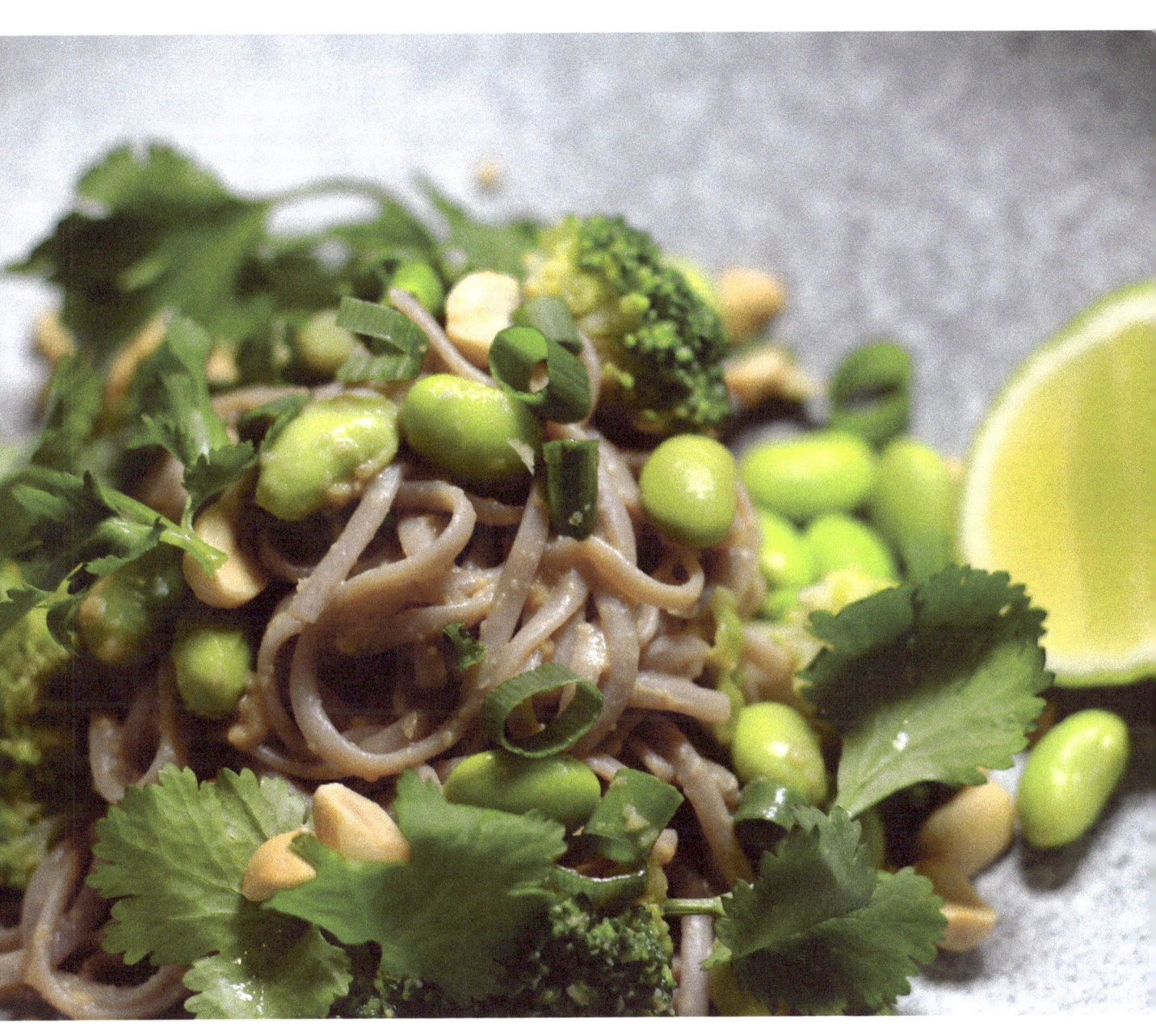

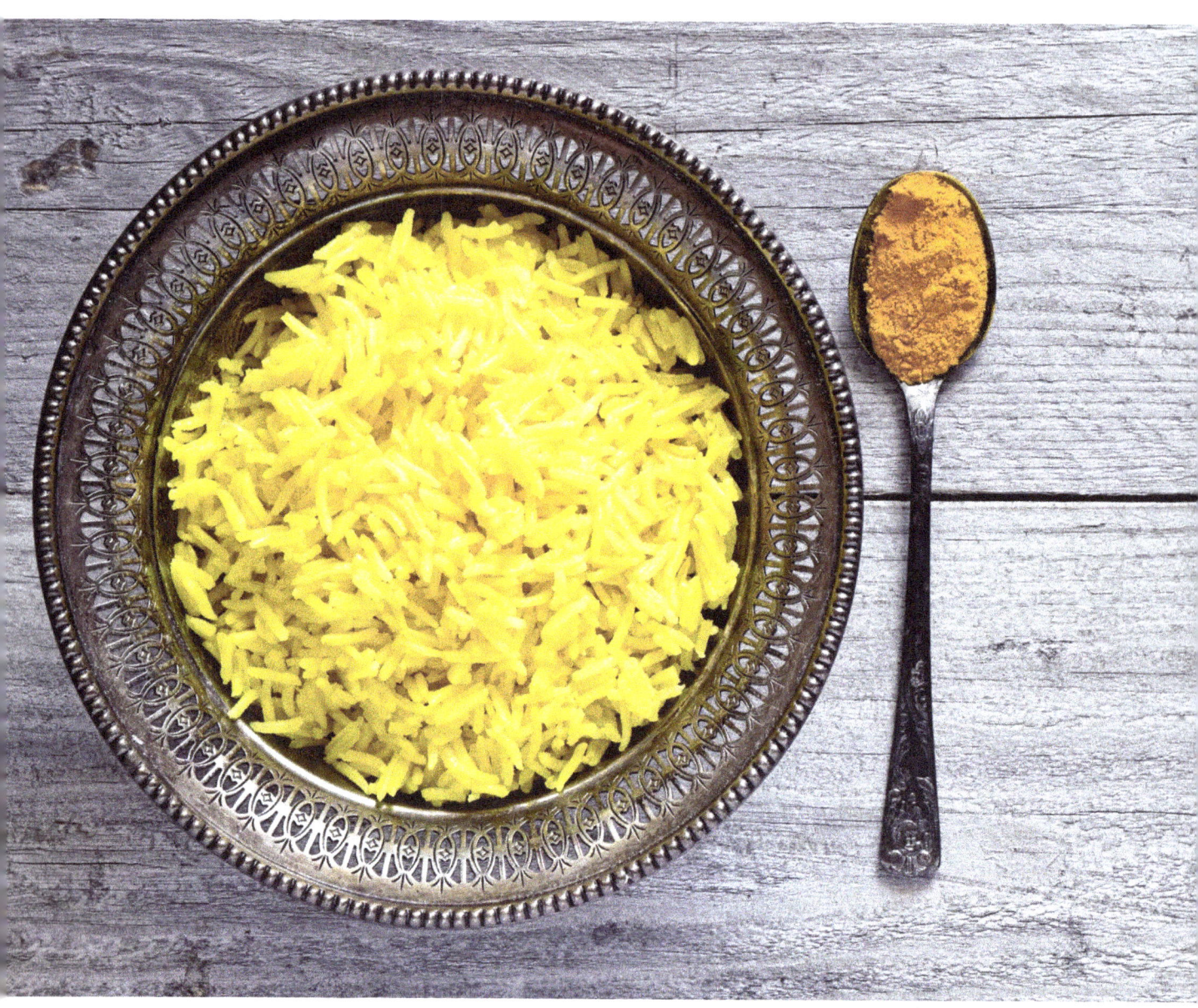

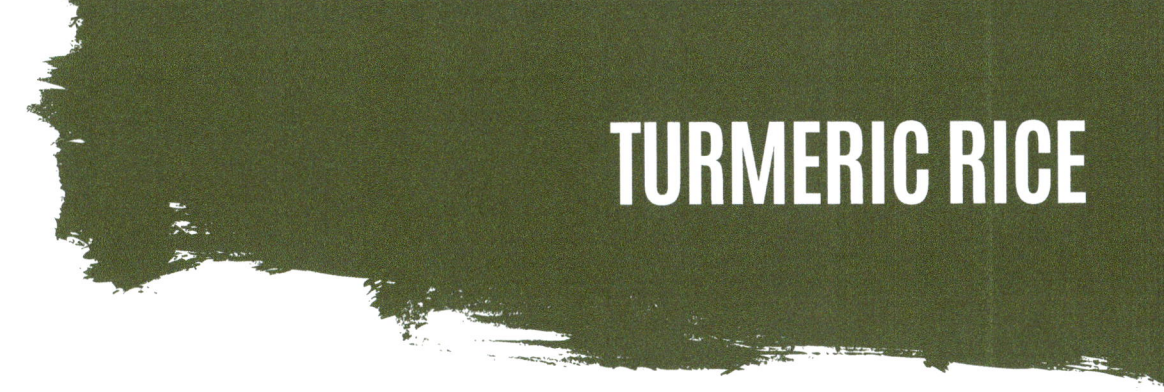

TURMERIC RICE

PREPARATION TIME
15 MINUTES

COOKING TIME
20 MINUTES

SERVES
4

INGREDIENTS:

30ml garlic infused olive oil
1 finely diced celery stick
200gm basmati rice
10gm turmeric
375ml vegetable broth
1 bay leaf
1gm dried thyme
salt and pepper to taste

METHOD:

1. In a medium saucepan add 15ml of the oil and place over medium heat.
2. Once hot, add finely diced celery and cook until softened.
3. Add rice and turmeric and stir to coat.
4. Add remaining ingredients, bring to the boil, cover and simmer 15 minutes.
5. Stir in remaining oil, remove bay leaf, serve.

This can be used as a salad, a side or an easy Friday night dinner. Just add steamed vegetables to bulk it up. It is lovely with a marinated tofu steak and a side of greens.

ZUCCHINI AND HAZELNUT SALAD WITH WALNUT VINAIGRETTE

PREPARATION TIME
20 MINUTES

COOKING TIME
20 MINUTES

SERVES
6

INGREDIENTS:

600gm zucchini
100gm hazelnuts
120gm rocket
Macadamia feta
Salt and pepper to taste
1 serve walnut vinaigrette, recipe found on page 144
Garlic infused olive oil for brushing the zucchini

METHOD:

1. Using a mandolin or vegetable peeler, slice the zucchini lengthways or crossways.
2. Lightly brush both sides of the zucchini with the garlic infused olive oil.
3. On a large French grill, fry both sides of the zucchini until lightly charred. Season to taste and set aside.
4. Roughly chop the hazelnuts and place in the fry pan and gently dry fry for 2 minutes until golden.
5. Place the rocket on a serving dish. Arrange half the charred zucchini over the rocket. Sprinkle with half the crushed hazelnuts.
6. Place remaining zucchini on top, sprinkle with remaining hazelnuts.
7. Scatter the feta over the top and around the zucchini and drizzle with the walnut vinaigrette.

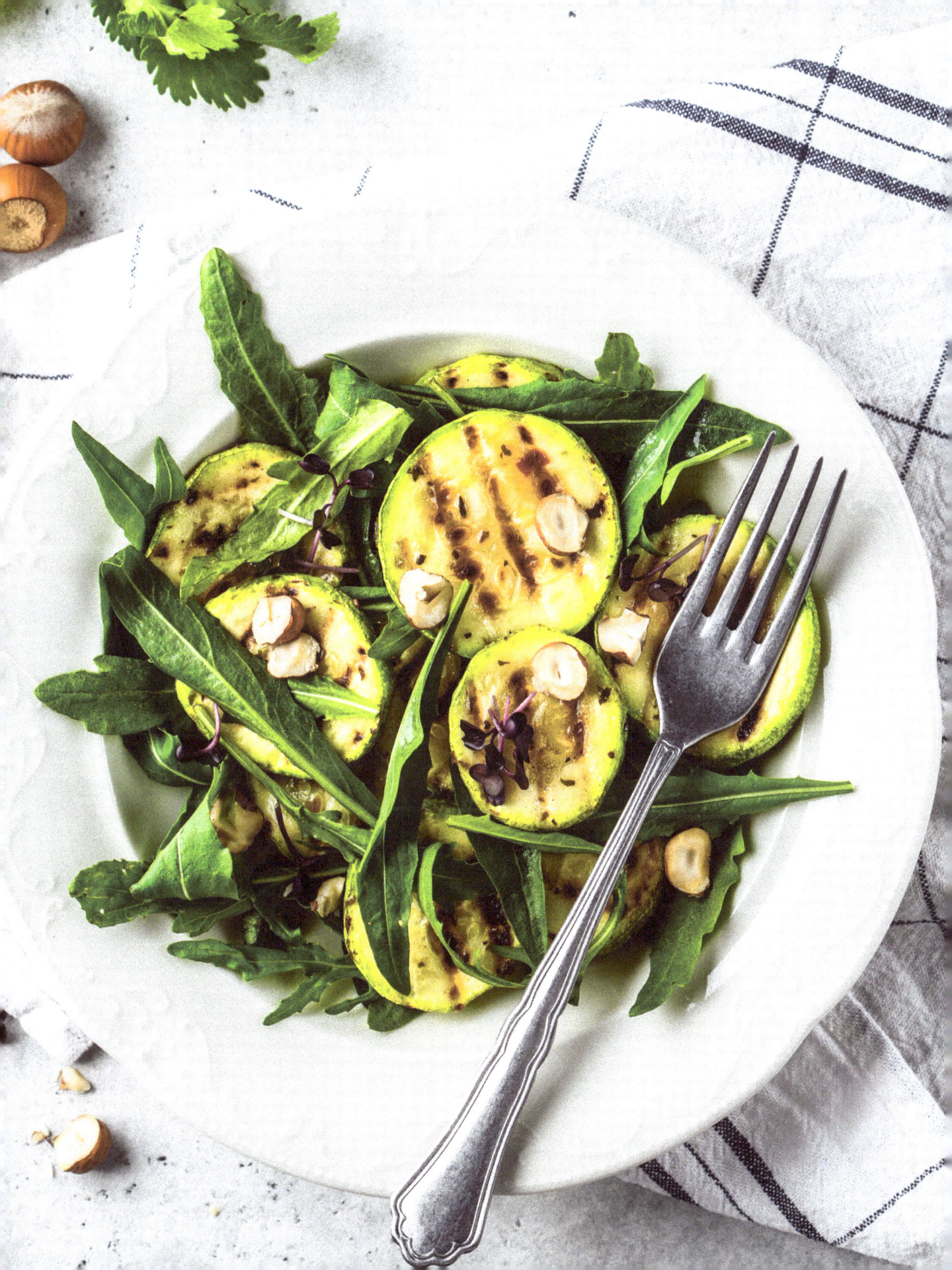

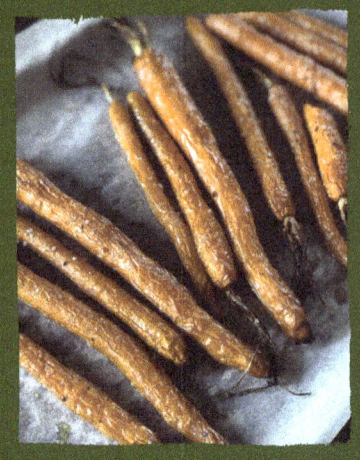
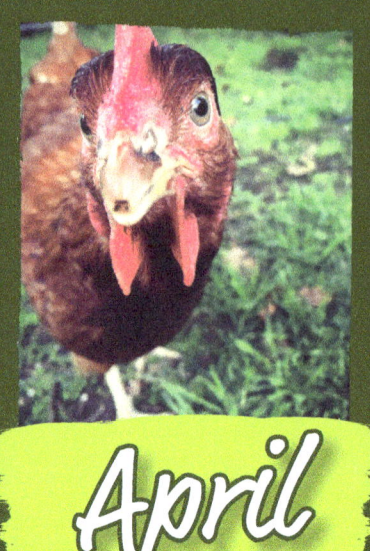
April
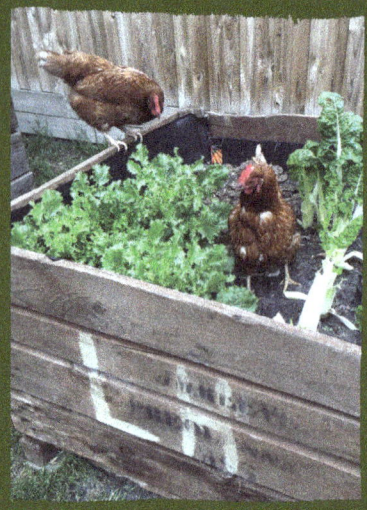

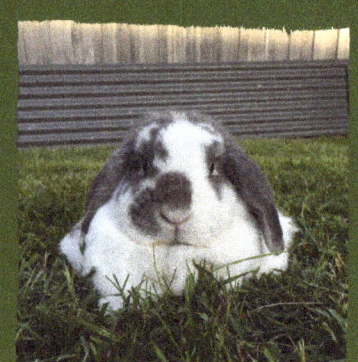
Luci
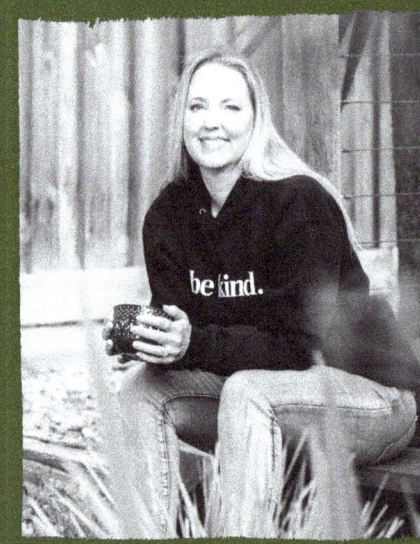
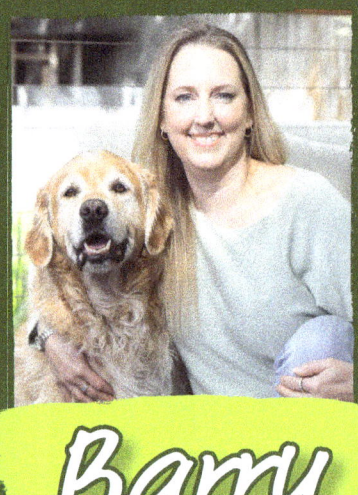
Barry

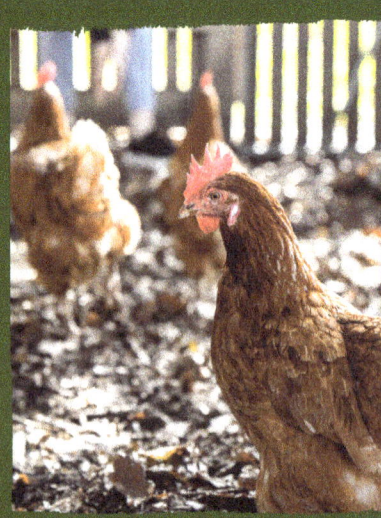
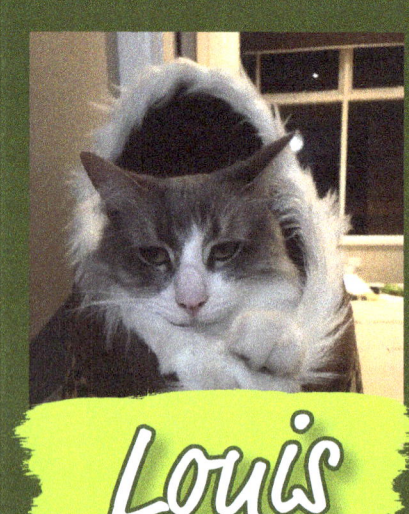
Louis
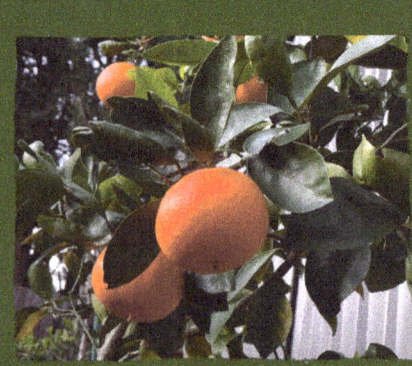

CHAPTER 4
Starters and Snacks

"Today be thankful and think how rich you are. Your family is priceless, your time is gold, and your health is wealth."
— Anonymous

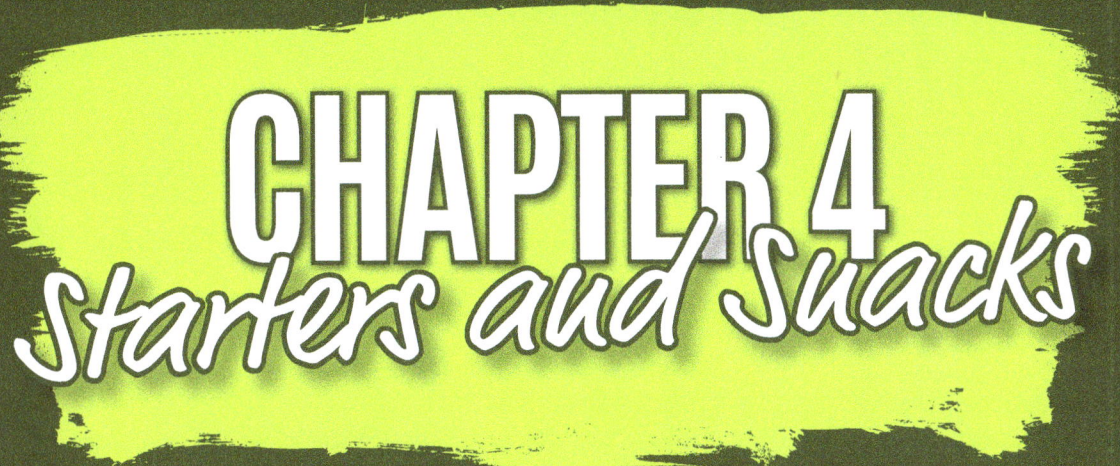

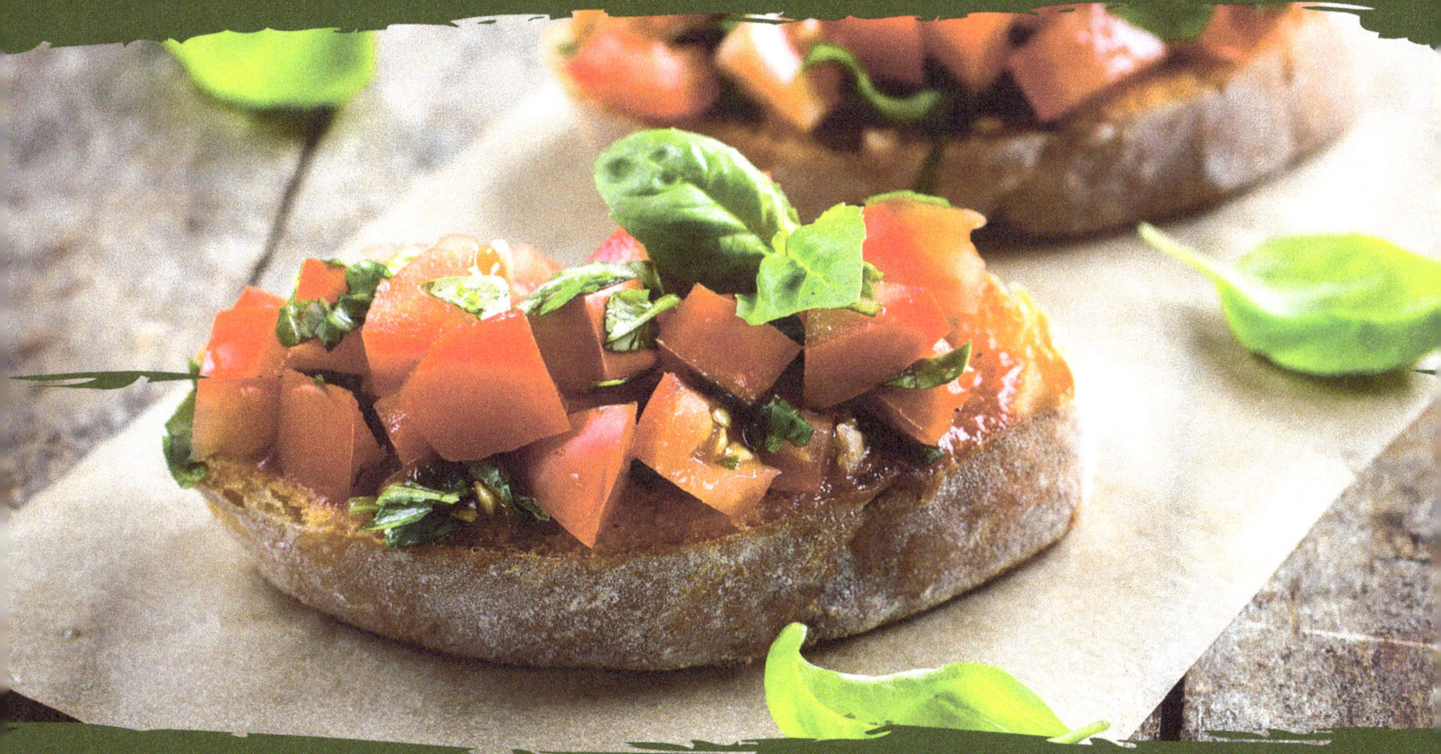

Whether we are entertaining or just having a relaxing day at home, everyone loves a snack or standing around a share platter with friends. Socialising is very much the Aussie way with family and friends being an integral part of our fabric. The following sides will get the juices dripping and the conversation flowing.

SPINACH EMPANADAS

PREPARATION TIME
45 MINUTES

COOKING TIME
20 MINUTES

SERVES
24

INGREDIENTS:

6 sheets of GF short crust pastry
Filling
1 bunch silverbeet
50gm pinenuts
50gm savoury yeast flakes
65gm vegan sour cream
Garlic infused oil for frying
S&P to taste
Black cumin seeds for sprinkling (optional)
Turmeric for sprinkling
Plant based milk for pastry

METHOD:

1. Preheat oven to 200°C.
2. Thoroughly wash spinach leaves.
3. Cut stems from silverbeet and dice thoroughly.
4. Roughly chop the leaves.
5. In a fry pan with lid, place enough oil in bottom and heat.
6. Once oil is hot, add diced spinach stems and fry until softened.
7. Once soft, add remaining chopped spinach.
8. Reduce heat, add a little water for steaming effect, place lid on and cook until wilted.
9. Once well wilted strain in colander, set aside and let cool.
10. In a small clean fry pan, lightly dry fry pinenuts until just golden brown.
11. Place pinenuts in a bowl with remaining ingredients and gently stir until thoroughly blended.
12. Squeeze excess water from cooled spinach and add to bowl. Mix thoroughly.

TO ASSEMBLE:

Using a 10cm cookie cutter, cut 4 rounds of pastry from the first sheet.

Place 1tsp of the mix into the centre of the pastry sheet.

With fingertip, place a little milk along one side of the pastry sheet.

Fold pastry over to surround the spinach mix and gently press edges together.

Place on lined cooking tray and press edges gently into the tray to give the classic empanada look…

Milk wash top of empanada and sprinkle with turmeric for a golden glow and/or black cumin seeds.

Bake for approximately 15–20 minutes or until golden brown.

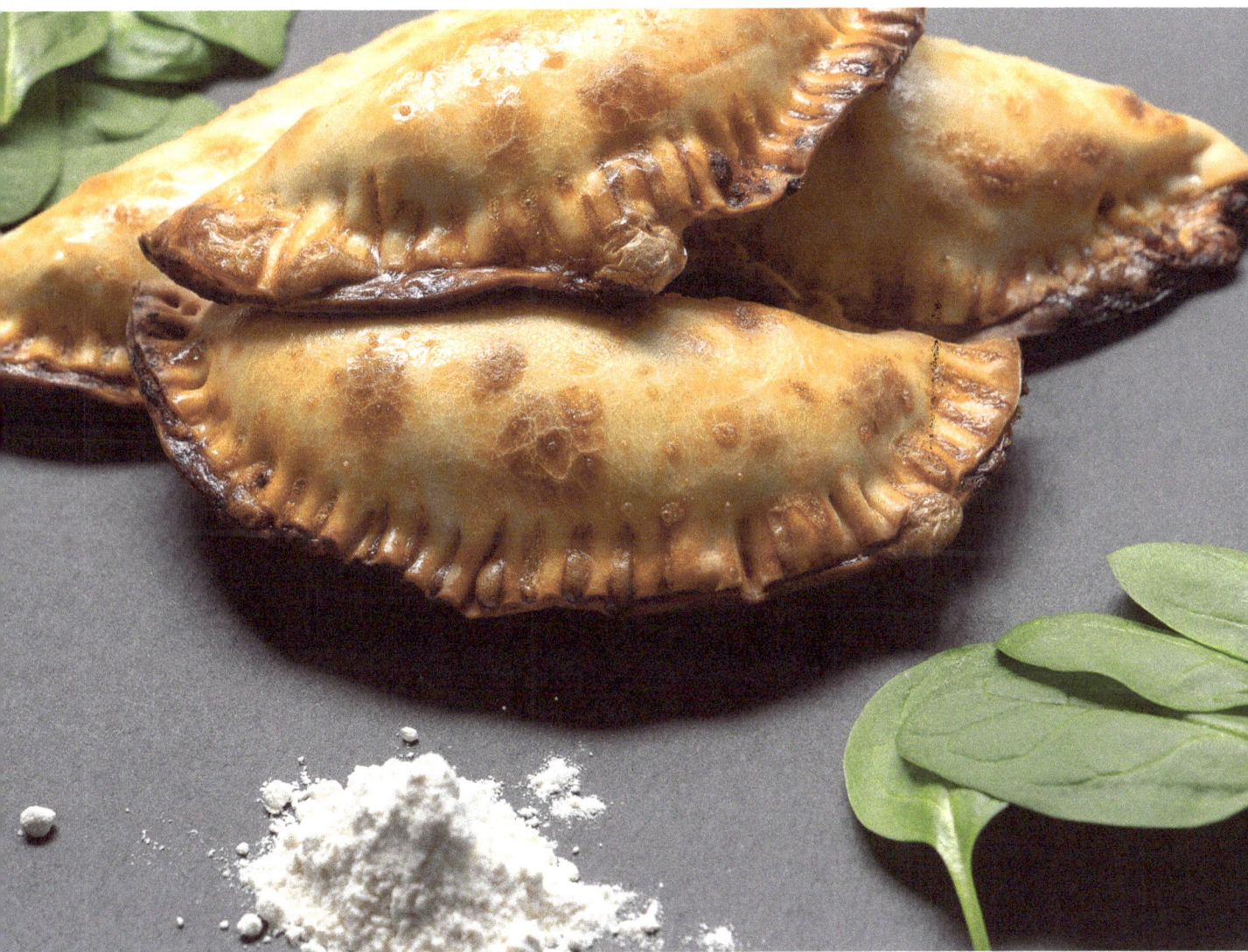

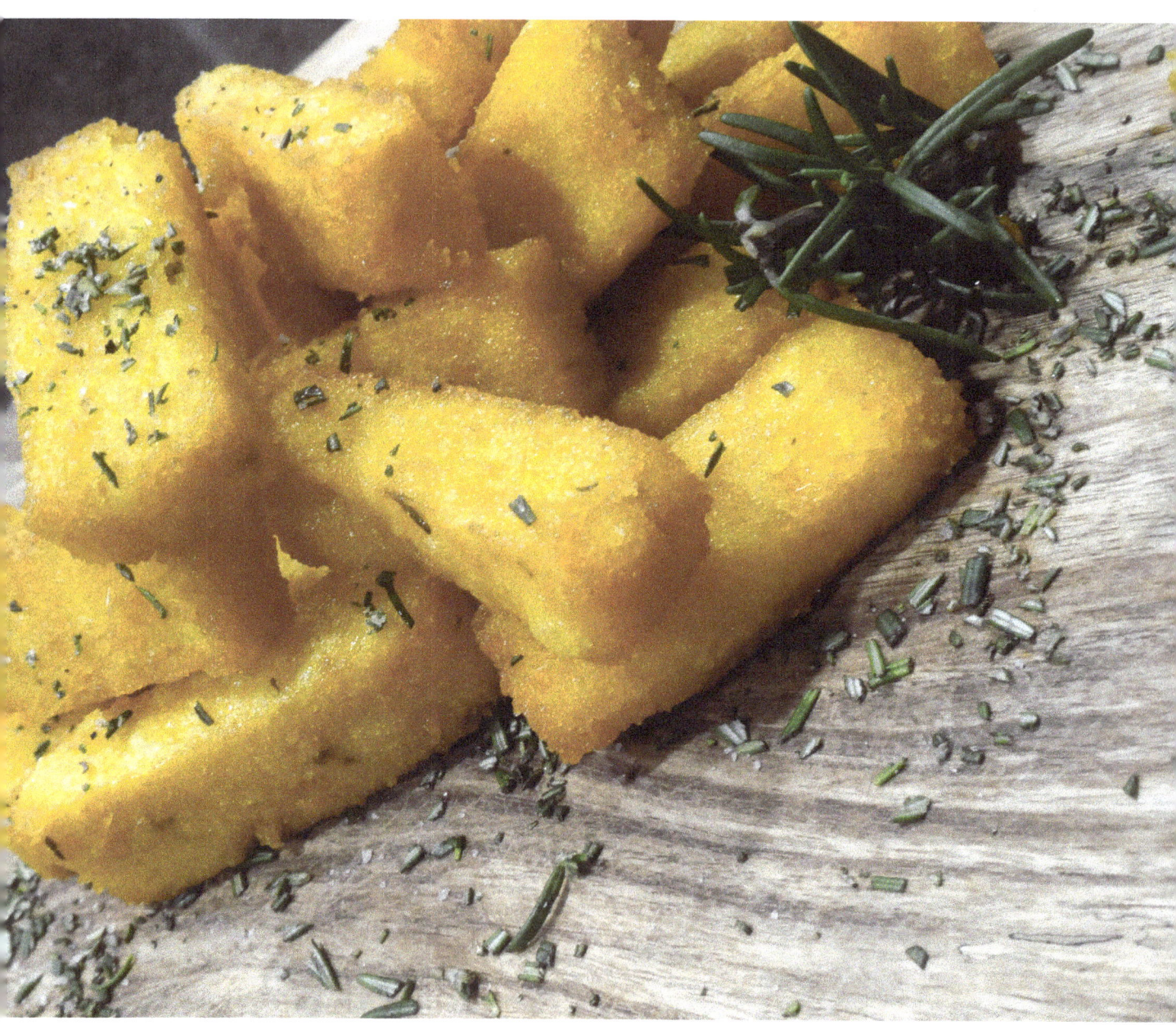

ROSEMARY POLENTA CHIPS

My family adores these. Overall, they are failproof and the recipe makes a lot – so plenty to share around. Although I don't believe they need anything other than the rosemary salt, you could try serving with some aioli. Make sure you are hungry as one is definitely not enough…

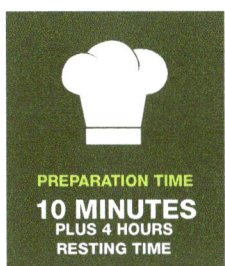

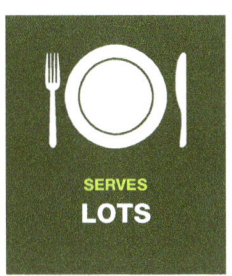

PREPARATION TIME
10 MINUTES PLUS 4 HOURS RESTING TIME

COOKING TIME
5 MINUTES EACH

SERVES
LOTS

INGREDIENTS:

8 cups water
10gm Himalayan sea salt
500gm instant GF fine polenta
2gm dry Italian herbs
40gm savoury yeast flakes
½ bunch rosemary, leaves removed from woody stems
Extra 10gm Himalayan sea salt

METHOD:

1. Line a 15x30cm baking tray with baking paper.
2. Bring water and salt to the boil.
3. Using a wooden spoon, add polenta and herbs whisking until all thoroughly combined and no lumps are visible.
4. Taking polenta off the heat, add the SYF and blend thoroughly.
5. Pour hot mixture onto the lined tray and flatten with a wet wooden spoon.
6. Let cool – refrigerate approx. 4 hours or overnight.

Cut to desired chip length and deep fry in ricebran oil.

To serve, chop fresh rosemary with Himalayan sea salt on a wooden board to season it. Keep a little to the side to sprinkle over the chips.

Place chips on the seasoned board and drizzle with olive oil. Eat by rolling the chips in the rosemary/salt blend.

NUT FETA STUFFED ZUCCHINI FLOWERS

PREPARATION TIME
45 MINUTES

COOKING TIME
5 MINUTES EACH

SERVES
20

INGREDIENTS:

Zucchini flowers
1 batch macadamia feta
15gm fresh basil leaves
1gm chilli flakes
120gm plain GF flour
125gm tapioca flour
4gm Himalayan sea salt
2gm black cracked pepper
1.5gm paprika
500ml water – more if required
Ricebran oil for deep frying

METHOD:

1. Blend feta, finely chopped basil leaves and chilli flakes together.
2. Pull stamen out of each flower.
3. Place mixture into a piping bag and fill inside the flowers until plump. Placing leaves back over the feta filling so you don't see the mixture.
4. Place in fridge at least 1 hour to set.
5. Place flours, salt, pepper, paprika and water in a bowl and whisk until well blended and quite a thin batter. Add more water if required.
6. Carefully dip the zucchini flowers into the batter and place into hot oil until browned.
7. These do not take long to cook, approx. 5 minutes tops

Makes approx. 20 flowers

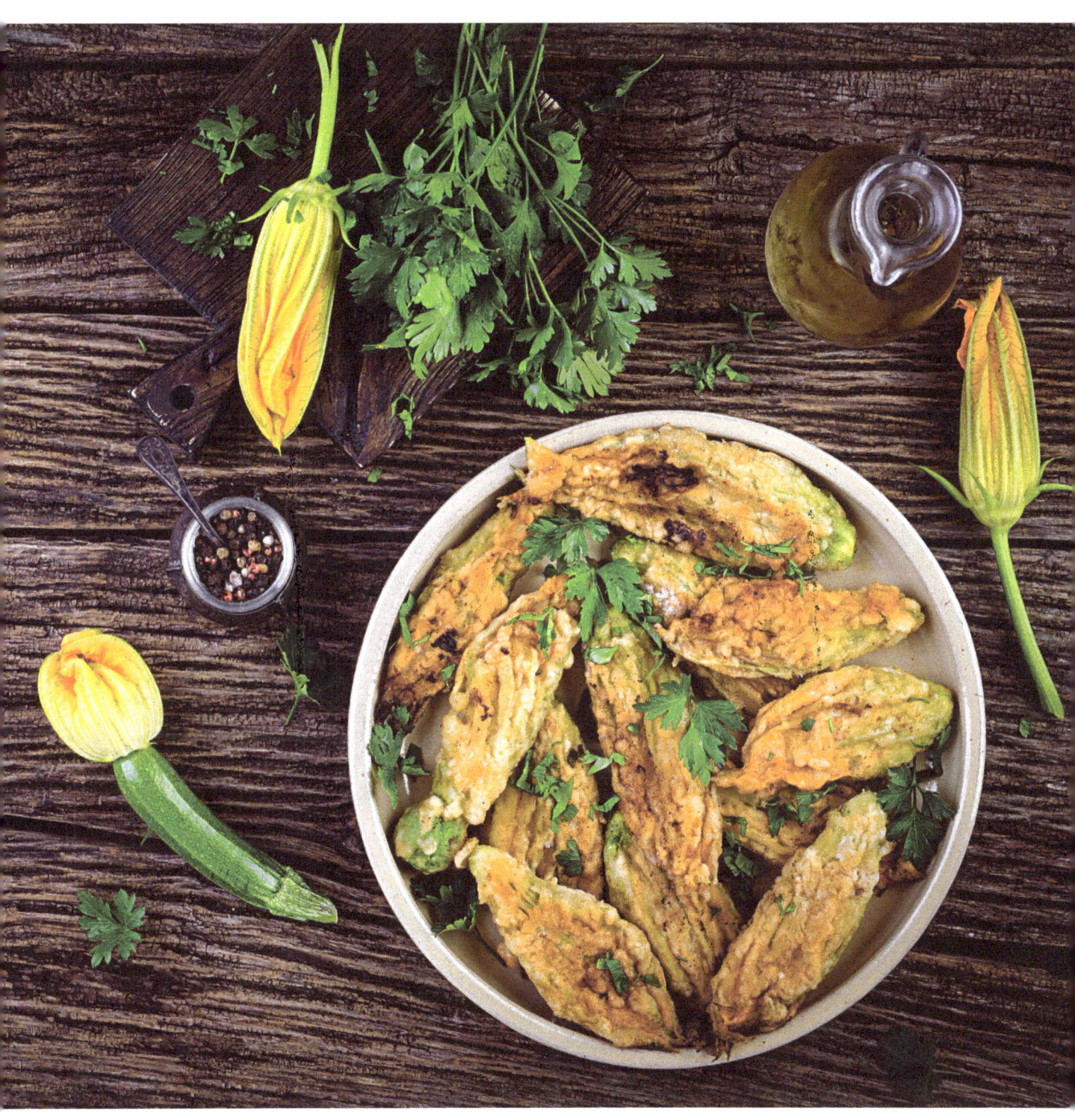

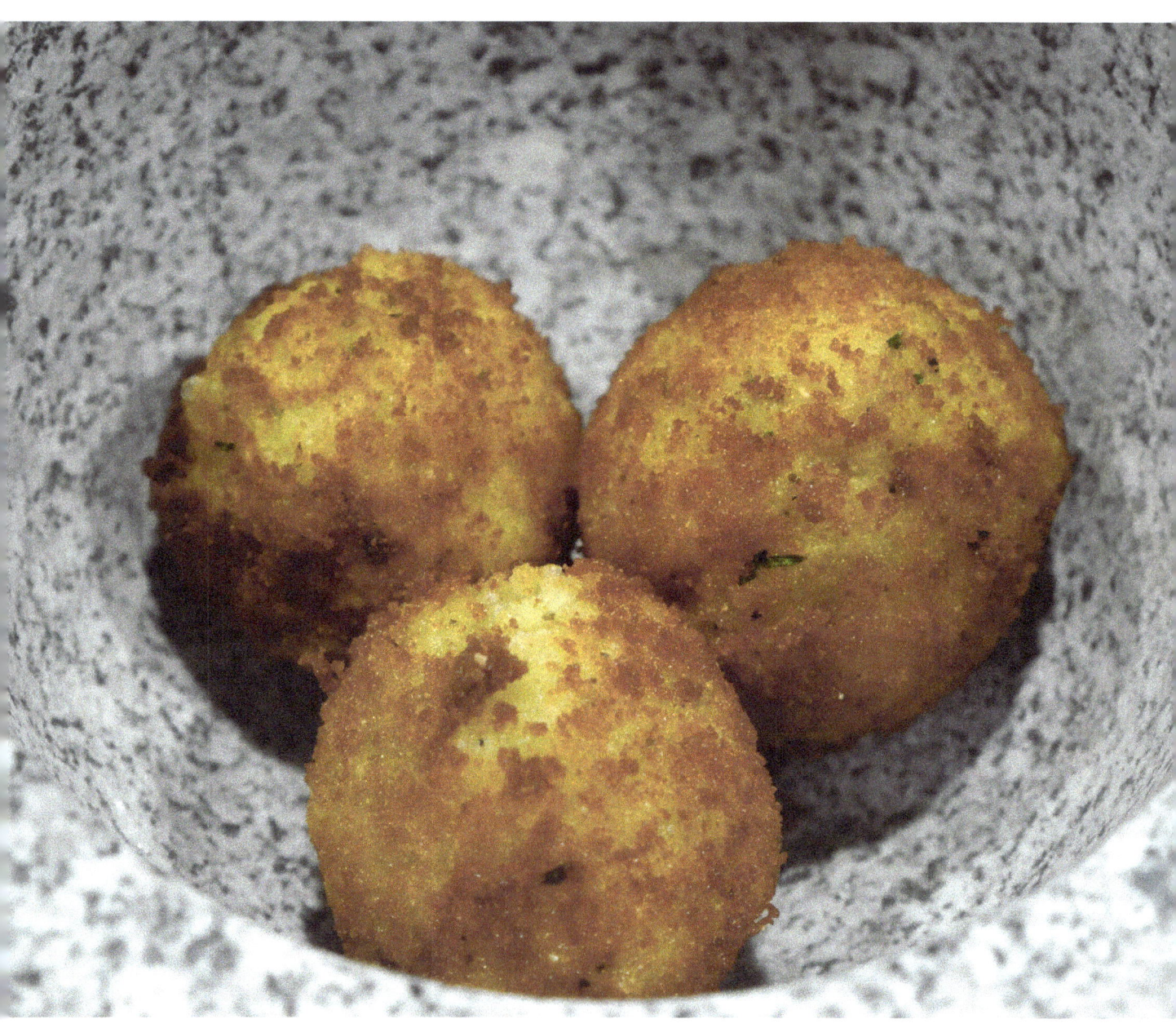

SUNDRIED TOMATO AND FETA ARANCINI BALLS

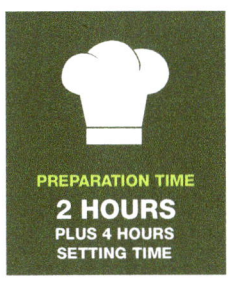
PREPARATION TIME
2 HOURS
PLUS 4 HOURS SETTING TIME

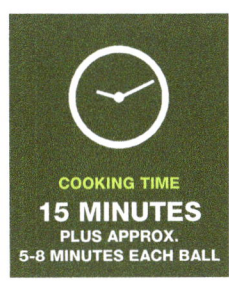
COOKING TIME
15 MINUTES
PLUS APPROX. 5-8 MINUTES EACH BALL

SERVES
18 BALLS

INGREDIENTS:

RICE
3 cups water
300gm Arborio rice
6gm Himalayan sea salt
20ml rice bran oil
10gm Himalayan sea salt
30gm savoury yeast flakes
2gm finely chopped basil leaves
20gm powdered egg replacer

FILLING
40gm semidried tomatoes – finely chopped
250gm macadamia feta cheese
4 sprigs freshly chopped parsley
Rice bran oil for shallow frying
Extra egg replacer for dipping
GF breadcrumbs for crumbing

VARIATION...

Also delicious when filled with:

Walnut bolognaise

Macadamia nut pesto

METHOD:

1. Blend feta, sundried tomatoes and parsley in a bowl, set aside.
2. Rinse rice under cold running water.
3. Place water, rice, 6gm salt and oil in a large saucepan.
4. Bring to the boil, reduce heat, cover with lid and let simmer for 15 minutes.
5. Once cooked, turn off heat, leave the lid on and let sit for 5 minutes to complete absorption of fluid.
6. Once ready, fluff with a fork and place into a large bowl.
7. While rice is still hot, add remaining salt, savoury yeast flakes, basil and egg replacer.
8. Keeping hands wet and working with a hot mix, take approx. 40gm scoop of rice, mould into palm of hand making a well in centre of rice mix.
9. Take 1 tsp of feta mix and place in well, gently surrounding feta mix with rice until a ball is formed.
10. Continue until all balls are formed and refrigerate minimum 4 hours or until set firmly.
11. Make up egg replacer according to directions.
12. Dip balls into the egg mix until totally covered then proceed to dip into the breadcrumbs.
13. Refrigerate for minimum 1 hour.
14. Heat oil and fry until golden brown.

Jodie Martin | **Chapter 4** Starters and Snacks

CUCUMBER BITES

**PREPARATION TIME
10 MINUTES**

INGREDIENTS:

2 Lebanese cucumbers
Macadamia feta
Roasted capsicum strips
Semidried tomatoes

METHOD:

1. Wash and dry cucumbers.
2. Cut into 1cm widths.
3. Top with
    - Feta, roasted capsicum sliver.
    - Feta, semidried tomato sliver.
    - No-egg salad.
    - Chickpea tuna.
    - 5gm avocado, hemp seeds and squeeze lime juice.

You are limited only by your imagination with these cucumber rounds.

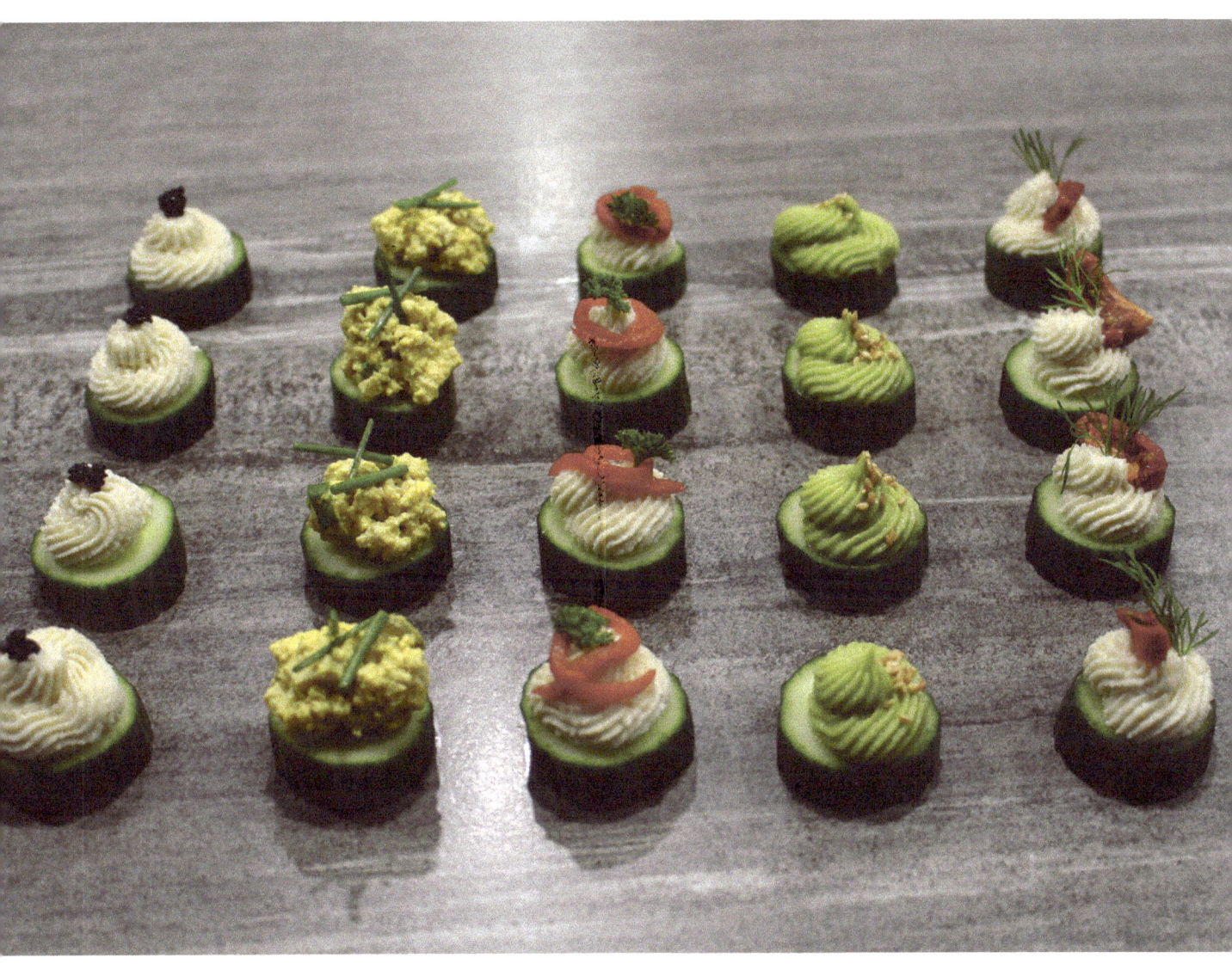

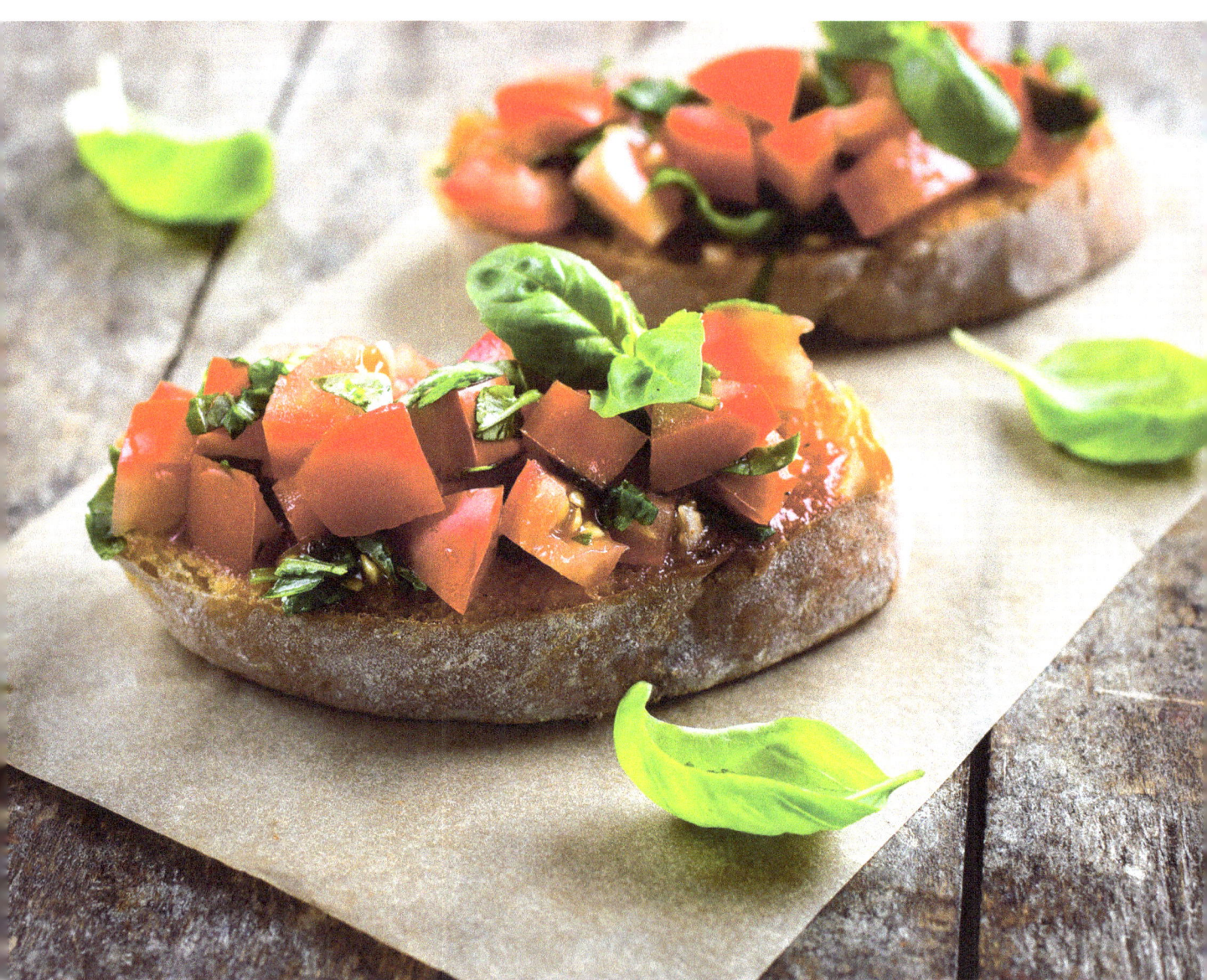

BRUSCHETTA

PREPARATION TIME: 20 MINUTES

COOKING TIME: 8 MINUTES

INGREDIENTS:

1 GF bread stick//baguette
Garlic infused olive oil
2-3 tomatoes deseeded and diced
Fresh basil, washed thoroughly
Salt and black cracked pepper to taste

METHOD:

1. Preheat oven to 180°C.
2. Slice bread stick into 1cm slices. Brush both sides with oil.
3. Place on a lined baking tray and bake for 6-8 minutes, until starting to brown.
4. Remove from oven.
5. Place diced tomatoes and picked leaves of basil into a bowl, drizzle with oil and season to taste.
6. Divide tomato mix evenly over the bread. Decorate with small leaves of basil.
7. To add extra deliciousness, you can add a sprinkle of feta.

OLIVE TAPENADE

INGREDIENTS:

2 cups pitted black kalamata olives
8gm fresh parsley
2.5gm fresh thyme
100ml garlic infused olive oil
(plain olive oil can be used also)
Black cracked pepper to taste
Squeeze lemon juice to taste

METHOD:

Place all ingredients in a blender and blitz until desired consistency.

This can be served as a dip with vegetable batons or spread on a crunchy baguette with finger lime caviar.

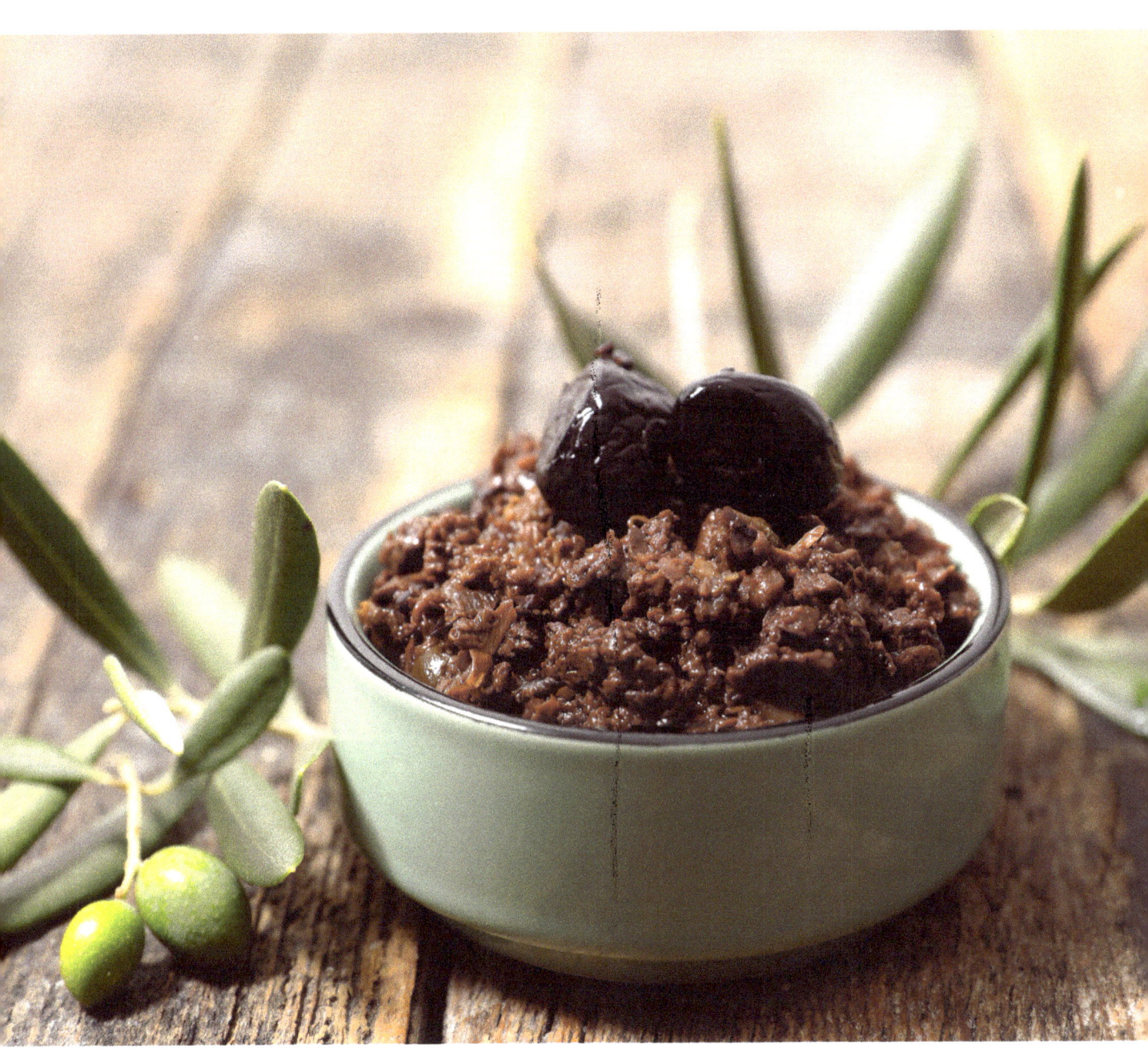

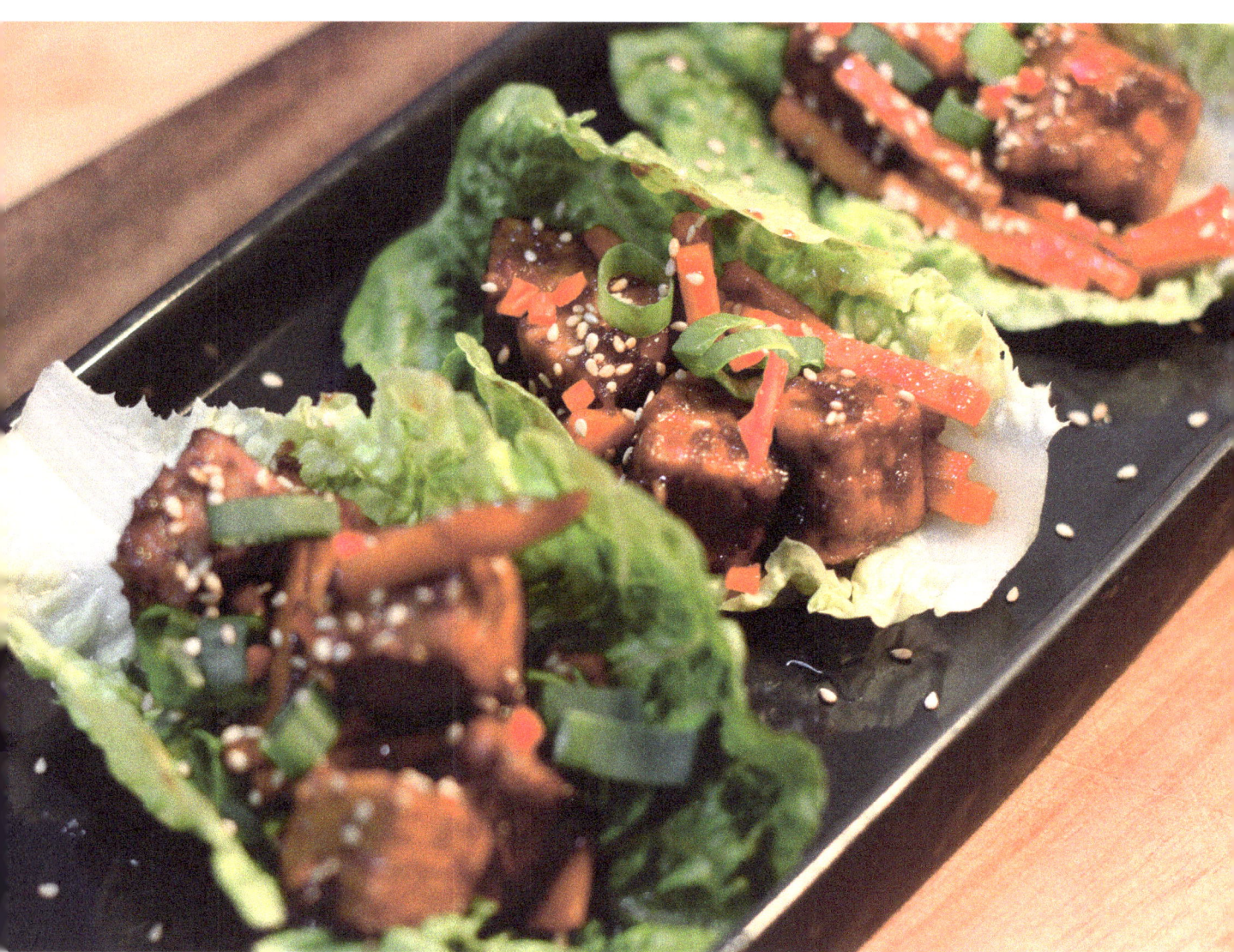

STICKY TEMPEH LETTUCE BOAT

PREPARATION TIME
5 MINUTES

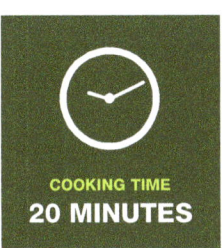
COOKING TIME
20 MINUTES

SERVES
3

INGREDIENTS:

1x 200gm tempeh, cut into 1cm cubes
45ml GF tamari
30ml lemon juice
5ml sesame oil
30ml 100% maple syrup
40gm crushed ginger
10ml garlic infused olive oil
2 medium carrots, cut into matchsticks
3 large cos lettuce leaves washed and allowed to dry off
2 spring onions, green tops only, finely sliced
10gm sesame seeds
2 small chillies, finely sliced (optional)

METHOD:

1. In a small bowl, mix the soy sauce, lemon juice, sesame oil, maple syrup, 1 chilli and ginger.

2. Add the tempeh and toss until tempeh is totally coated. Allow to sit as long as you can.

3. In a medium fry pan, add oil and place over medium heat. Add the tempeh along with excess marinade. Cook for about 10 minutes, turning as the liquid cooks off and the tempeh is browned on multiple sides.

4. Add the carrots. Increase heat to high and fry for about a minute or until the carrots are tender but still have a crunch.

5. Divide the mixture onto lettuce leaves and top with spring onions, remaining chilli and sesame seeds.

6. Enjoy.

SATAY TOFU SKEWERS

INGREDIENTS:

500gm firm tofu
300gm fresh peanuts
15ml garlic infused olive oil plus extra for the tofu
30ml peanut oil
½ chilli, finely chopped (optional)
10gm grated ginger
45ml tamari
400ml can coconut cream
30gm coconut sugar
Juice of ½ lime
Himalayan sea salt to taste
Wooden skewers

PREPARATION TIME 30 MINUTES

COOKING TIME 10 MINUTES

SERVES 10 SKEWERS

METHOD:

SATAY SAUCE

1. Soak wooden skewers in water and set aside.
2. Add oils and peanuts in a fry pan and place over medium heat.
3. Once hot, add chilli and ginger and fry on a low heat until you can smell the fragrance and peanuts are light golden brown in colour.
4. Once cooked, allow to slightly cool. Place the peanuts in a blender and blitz until the mix resembles a rough crumb.
5. Return nut mix to the fry pan, heating them up and once hot, add coconut cream and sugar. Blend thoroughly.
6. Add tamari and mix thoroughly.
7. While stirring, slowly add the lime juice until desired flavour is reached. Keep tasting as you add the juice.
8. Add very slowly, as the mix can become over acidic if too much is added.
9. Add salt to taste.
10. This can be made ahead and stored in fridge. You can add more chilli, tamari or ginger according to taste. Adjust as required.

TOFU SKEWERS

1. Open and rinse tofu.
2. Cut into 1cm size squares.
3. Thread onto wooden skewers approx. 5 pieces each skewer.
4. Place some oil in a large fry pan.
5. Once hot, place skewers in fry pan/BBQ and cook until golden brown turning regularly.
6. Once cooked, place skewers on a serving dish and drizzle with satay sauce.
7. Excess sauce can be stored in fridge or frozen until needed.

If wanting to cook it the quick and easy way. Use 1 cup pure crunchy peanut butter.

1. Add chilli, ginger and oils in a medium saucepan.
2. Fry until fragrant.
3. Add the rest of the ingredients including the peanut butter to the saucepan and whisk continuously for several minutes until hot and smooth.
4. Pour over the skewers.

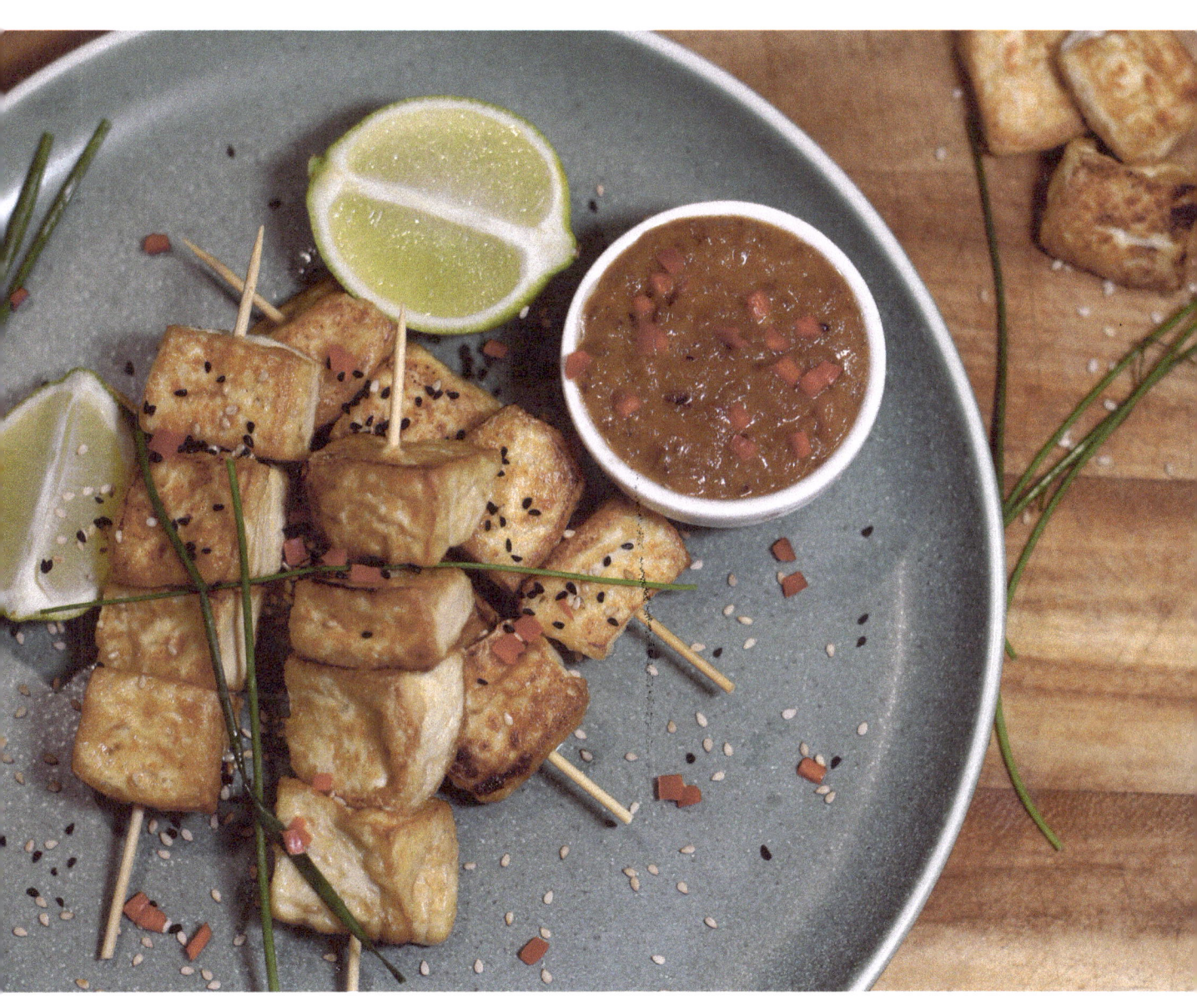

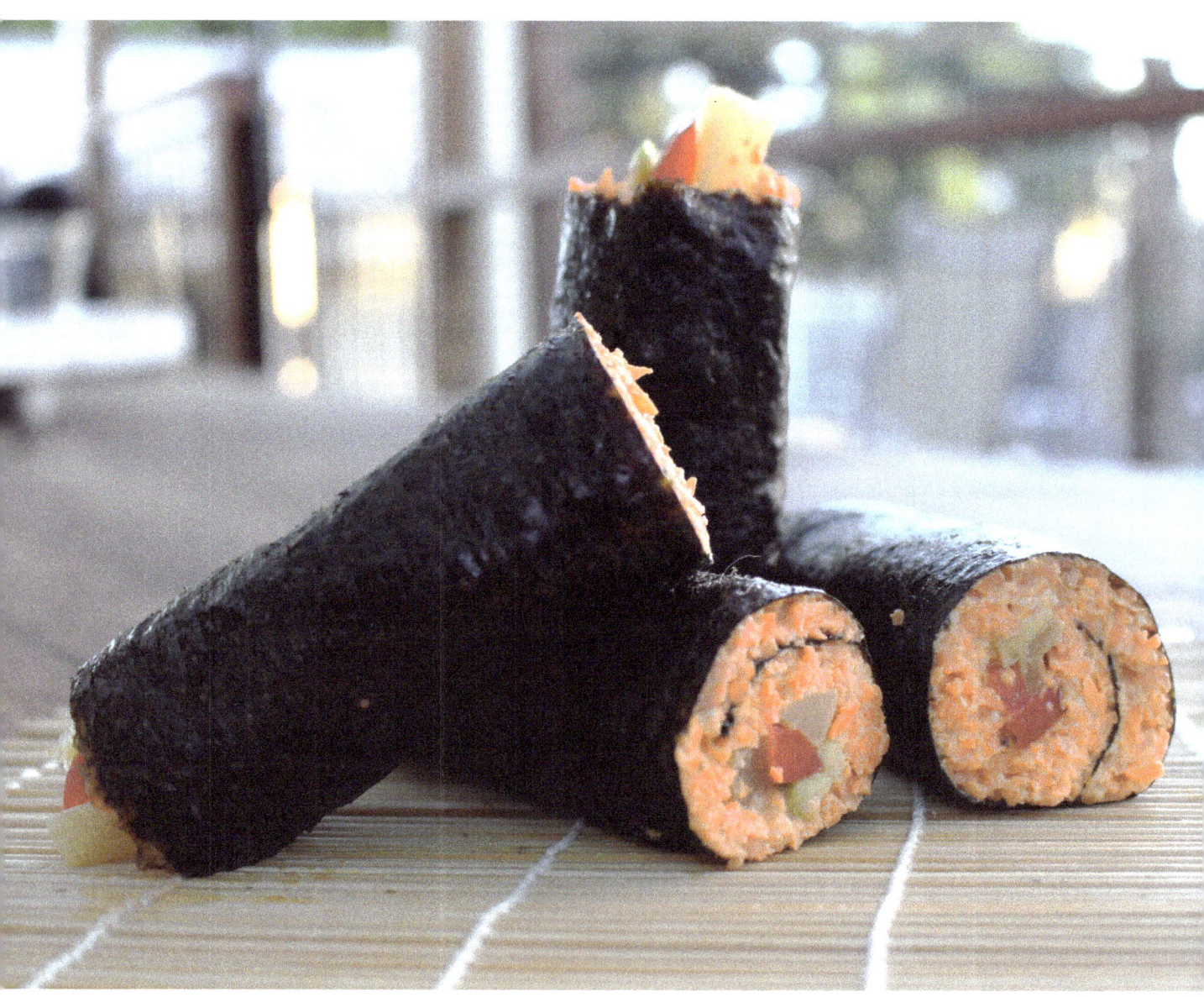

CARROT SUSHI

PREPARATION TIME
30 MINUTES

SERVES
2

INGREDIENTS:

4 carrots
125gm macadamia nut butter
10ml apple cider vinegar or rice wine vinegar
½ red capsicum, seeded and sliced into strips
75gm daikon radish, sliced into thin strips
20gm pickled ginger
60gm avocado
Vegan mayonnaise (optional)
Sesame seeds for sprinkling
2 nori sheets
Tamari for dipping
Nigella sativa seeds (optional)

METHOD:

1. Peel carrots and place in a food processor. Blitz until resembles a rice like texture.
2. Place in a bowl and add the ACV or rice wine vinegar and combine thoroughly. Let sit 5 minutes.
3. Add macadamia nut butter and blend thoroughly.
4. Place nori sheets on a clean bench, shiny side down.
5. Spread the carrot out evenly on both nori sheets leaving a border at one end approximately 3cm.
6. Place the vegetables along the bottom of the nori sheet, on top of the carrot rice.
7. Apply mayonnaise if required, down the side of the vegies.
8. Sprinkle with sesame seeds.
9. Rolling up from the vegie end, use your fingers and thumbs to keep it all intact, keeping it consistently tight.
10. Complete rolling to the end of the nori sheet.
11. Cut into 2-3 pieces with a sharp knife and enjoy with tamari.
12. Sprinkle with some extra black nigella sativa seeds for effect.

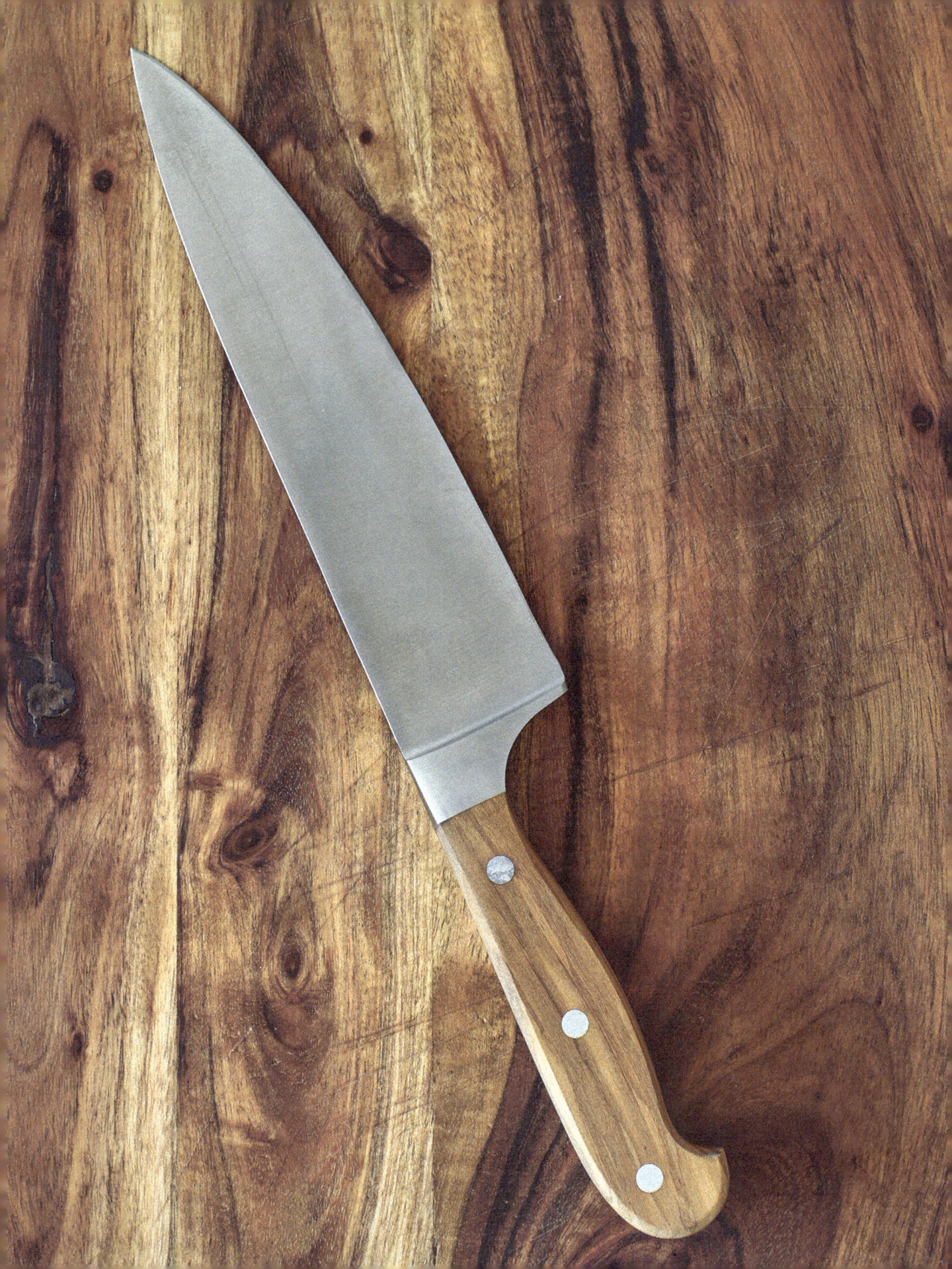

CHAPTER 5
Mains

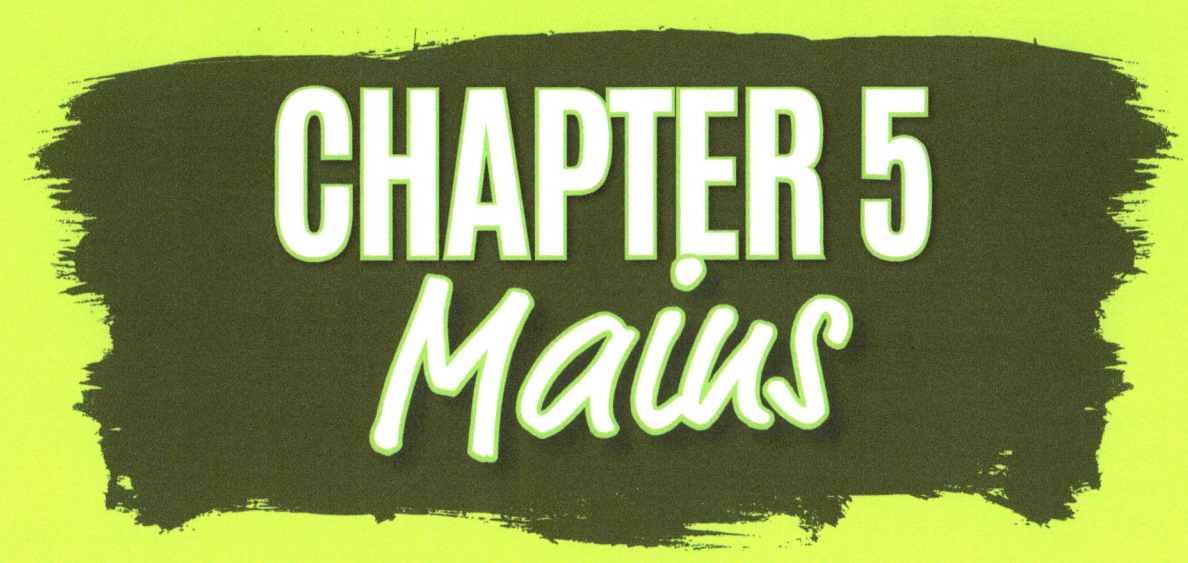

"I hold that the more helpless a creature, the more entitled it is to protection by man, from the cruelty of man."
– Mahatma Gandhi

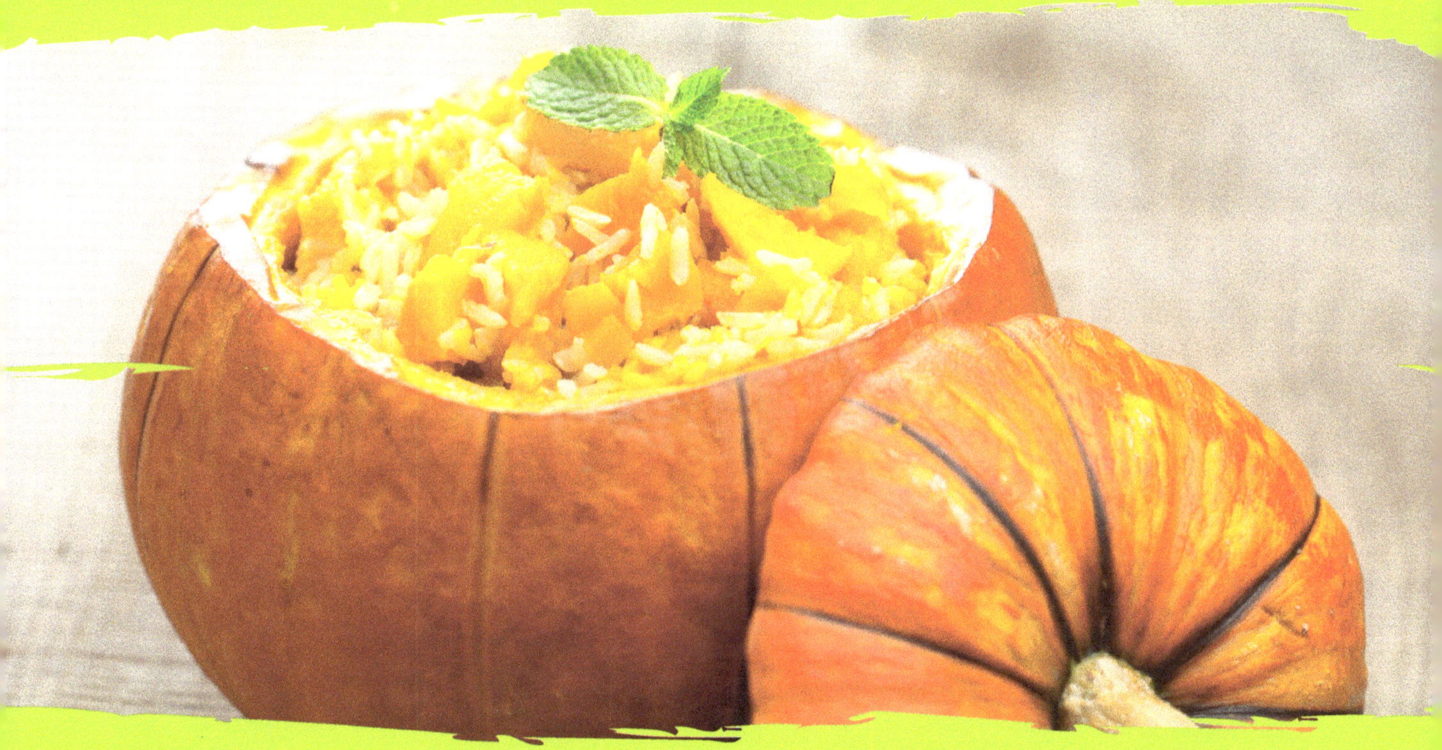

Dinner is my favourite meal of the day regardless of what the experts say!! I am controlled all day, but my willpower goes out the door at dinner time and I tend to enjoy more than my fair share. These are some of my family favourites and hope you enjoy them too.

WALNUT BOLOGNAISE

A different take on the usual meaty bolognaise sauce, this walnut bolognaise will give you the rich chewy feel you'd expect from a traditional 'bog'. It is rich and creamy, enjoy it thickly lathered over your pasta or you can try for a lighter option and add a dash of water to thin the sauce. Toss through your pasta/zucchini spirals.

PREPARATION TIME
10 MINUTES

COOKING TIME
15 MINUTES

SERVES
6

INGREDIENTS:

30ml garlic infused oil
130gm walnuts
15 semidried tomatoes
20gm SYF
50gm baby spinach leaves
– roughly chopped (optional)
1gm fresh oregano
1x 400gm can diced tomatoes
4gm coconut sugar
40gm tomato paste
Salt and pepper to taste
Dash of water to thin the sauce
4 medium zucchinis for spiralising or GF spaghetti pasta

METHOD:

1. Finely chop or blitz walnuts and semidried tomatoes.
2. Heat oil in a pan. Add walnuts and tomatoes and fry approx. 5 minutes.
3. Add diced tomatoes, oregano, SYF and coconut sugar and stir until thoroughly blended.
4. Add tomato paste and mix through thoroughly.
5. Add the water if required to thin the sauce.
6. Simmer 5 minutes.
7. Lastly add baby spinach if using and season to taste.
8. Spoon over GF spaghetti or zucchini spirals.

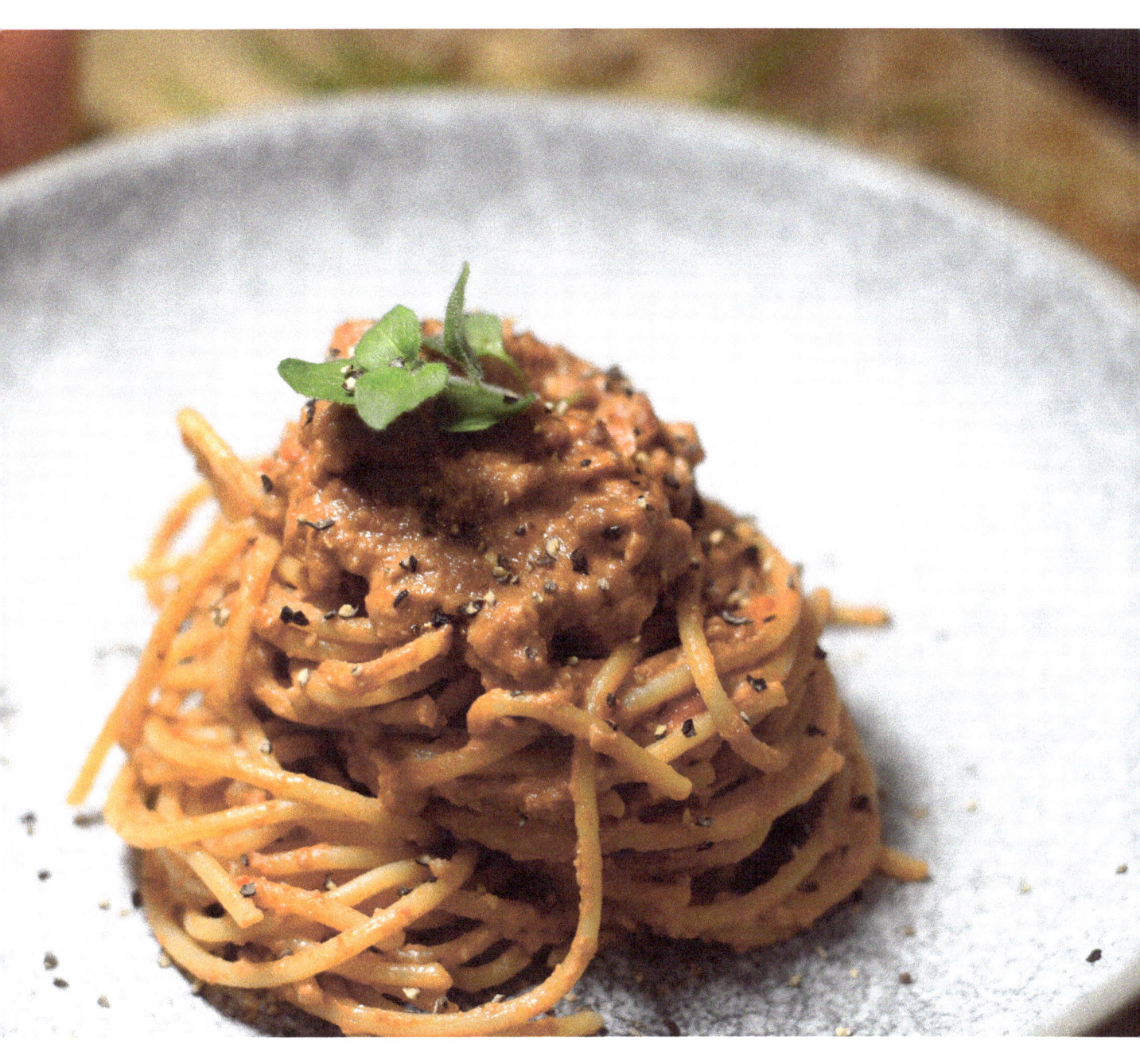

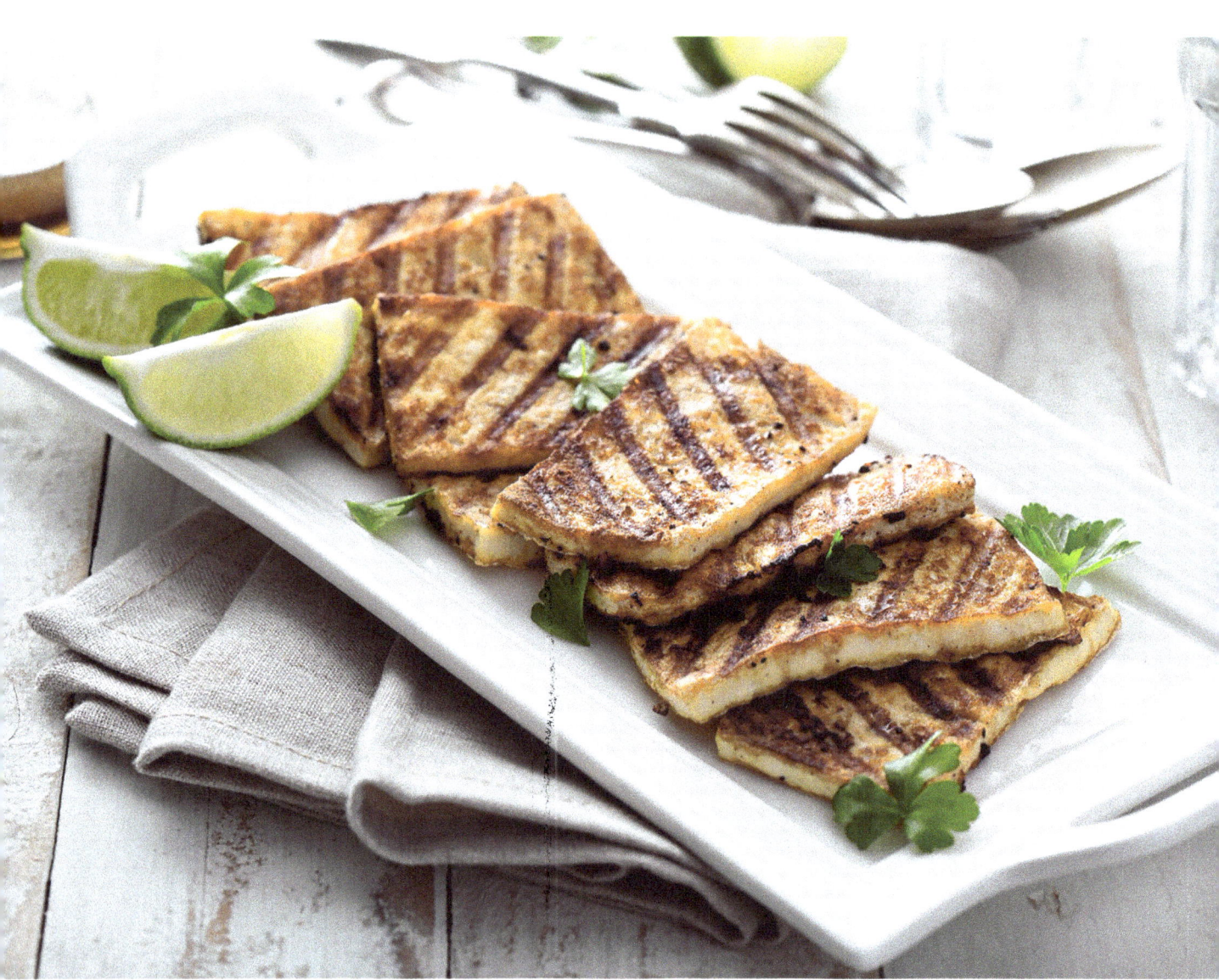

EASY PEASY TOFU STEAKS

PREPARATION TIME
15 MINUTES

COOKING TIME
10 MINUTES

SERVES
5

INGREDIENTS:

1x 500gm block firm tofu
1gm paprika
2gm turmeric
1gm cumin
Ricebran oil for shallow frying

METHOD:

1. Cut tofu into 1.5cm widths. Press in a tea towel to take some moisture out.
2. Blend paprika, turmeric and cumin.
3. Sprinkle over the tofu until well covered.
4. Heat oil in fry pan and shallow fry until golden brown.

These are great sliced and served in salads, served with vegies or in a salad sandwich.

MEXICAN TOFU STICKS

PREPARATION TIME
15 MINUTES

COOKING TIME
15 MINUTES

SERVES
6

INGREDIENTS:

10gm GF cornflour
1.5gm chilli powder
4gm Himalayan sea salt
2.5gm paprika
8gm brown sugar
3gm asafoetida (garlic type powder found in health food shops or Indian grocers)
0.5gm cayenne pepper
2.5gm ground cumin
2.5gm ground coriander
500gm block firm tofu
Ricebran oil for shallow frying

METHOD:

1. Cut tofu into 1cm wide strips.
2. Blend all dry ingredients and mix well.
3. Coat strips in the Mexican mix and shallow fry.

These go great in tacos, to dip in a chilli sauce or wraps with a salad.

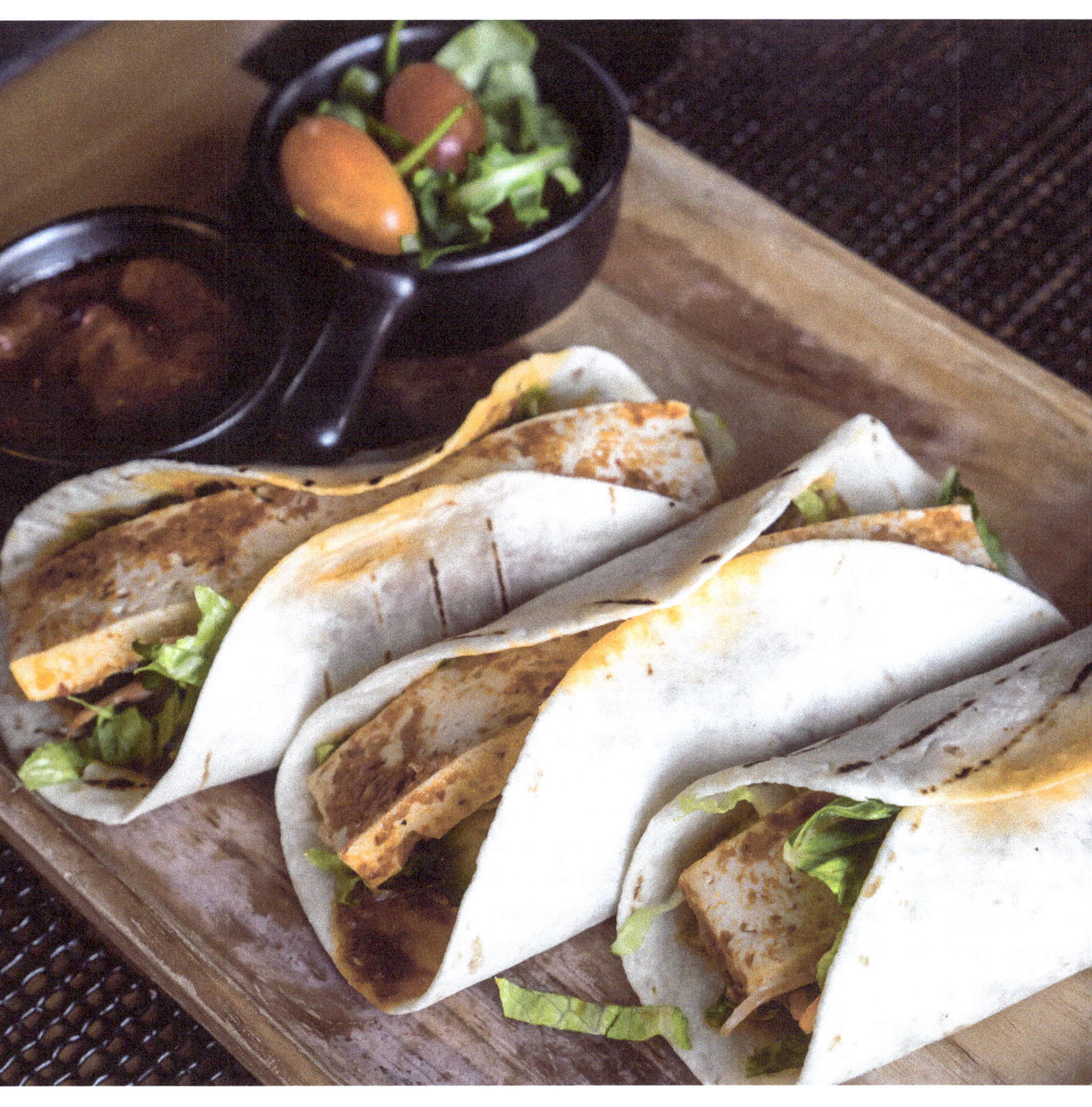

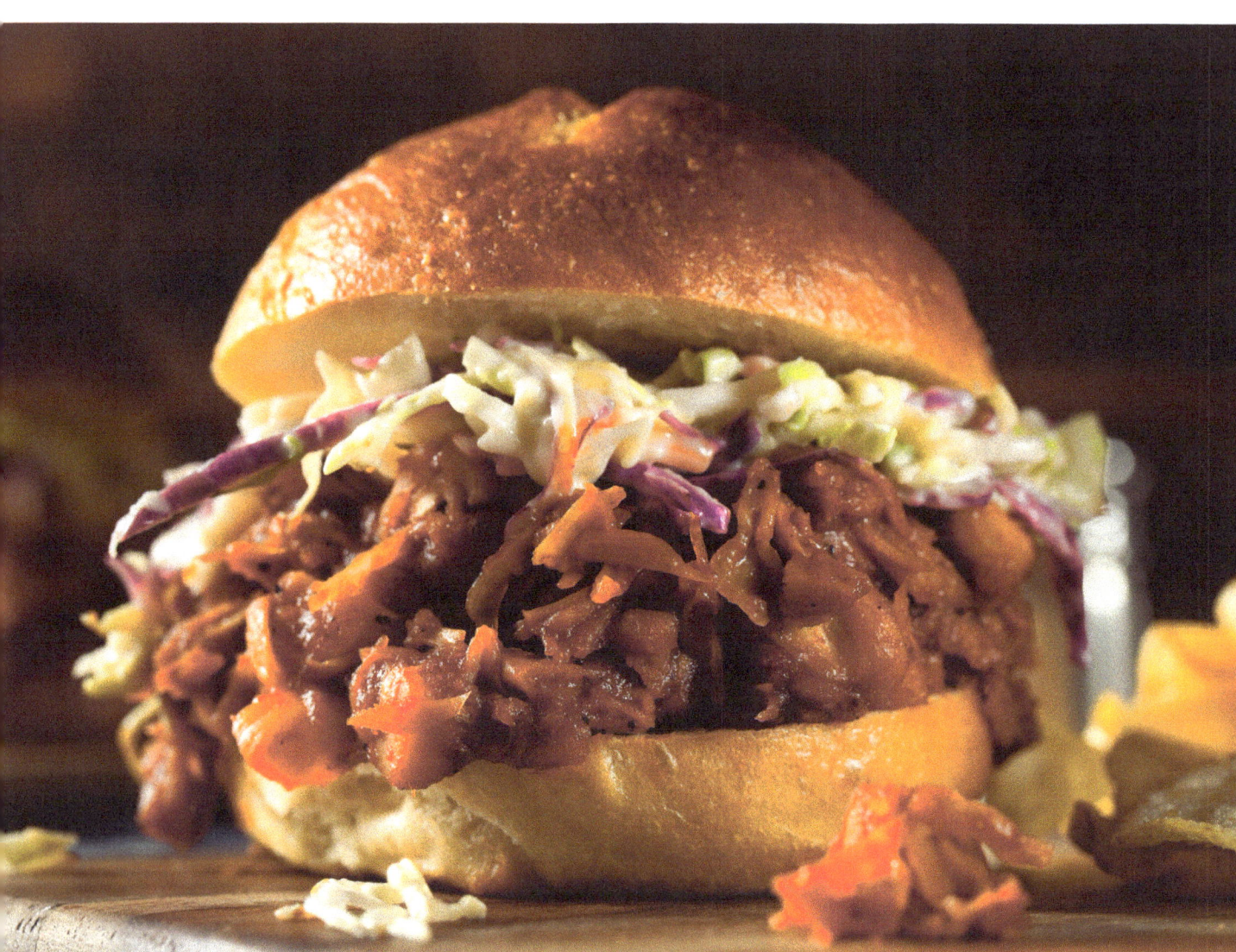

BBQ PULLED JACKFRUIT SLOPPY JOE

PREPARATION TIME
20 MINUTES

COOKING TIME
30 MINUTES

SERVES
8

INGREDIENTS:

2 400gm cans young jackfruit
60ml garlic infused olive oil
2 sticks celery
250ml water
1.5gm paprika
1gm cayenne pepper
2gm Himalayan sea salt

BBQ SAUCE
1 stick celery
30ml garlic infused olive oil
500ml tomato sauce
45gm coconut sugar
60ml tamari
60ml 100% maple syrup
40ml molasses
3gm fresh parsley (1gm dried)
3gm fresh thyme (1gm dried)
4gm Himalayan sea salt
8 GF hamburger buns

METHOD:

SAUCE

1. Heat oil in saucepan, add finely chopped celery.
2. Add remaining ingredients for the sauce and bring to boil.
3. Reduce heat and simmer 10 minutes or until sauce begins to thicken.
4. Drain jackfruit, pull it apart, roughly chop the core area and set aside. (The core and seeds cook quite soft so don't remove them.)
5. Heat oil in fry pan, add finely chopped celery and cook until starting to brown – approx. 5 minutes.
6. Stir in jackfruit and spices and mix to coat the jackfruit.
7. Add water and BBQ sauce to the jackfruit mix.
8. Simmer until sauce begins to thicken, approx. 3–5 mins.
9. Serve in a GF bread roll with coleslaw.

PUMPKIN RISOTTO

PREPARATION TIME
20 MINUTES

COOKING TIME
40 MINUTES

SERVES
4

INGREDIENTS:

250gm Kent or Queensland Blue pumpkin – diced
200gm arborio rice
1 stick celery
625ml hot low FODMAP vegetable stock
15gm vegan margarine
20gm savoury yeast flakes
½ bunch freshly chopped parsley
Large handful of baby spinach leaves (optional)
Salt and pepper to taste

METHOD:

1. Preheat oven 180°C.
2. Dice celery and pumpkin.
3. Place pumpkin, rice, celery, margarine and stock in an ovenproof dish.
4. Cover with lid, bake 30–40 minutes or until rice is tender.
5. Remove from oven, stir in savoury yeast flakes, baby spinach if using, parsley and season to taste.

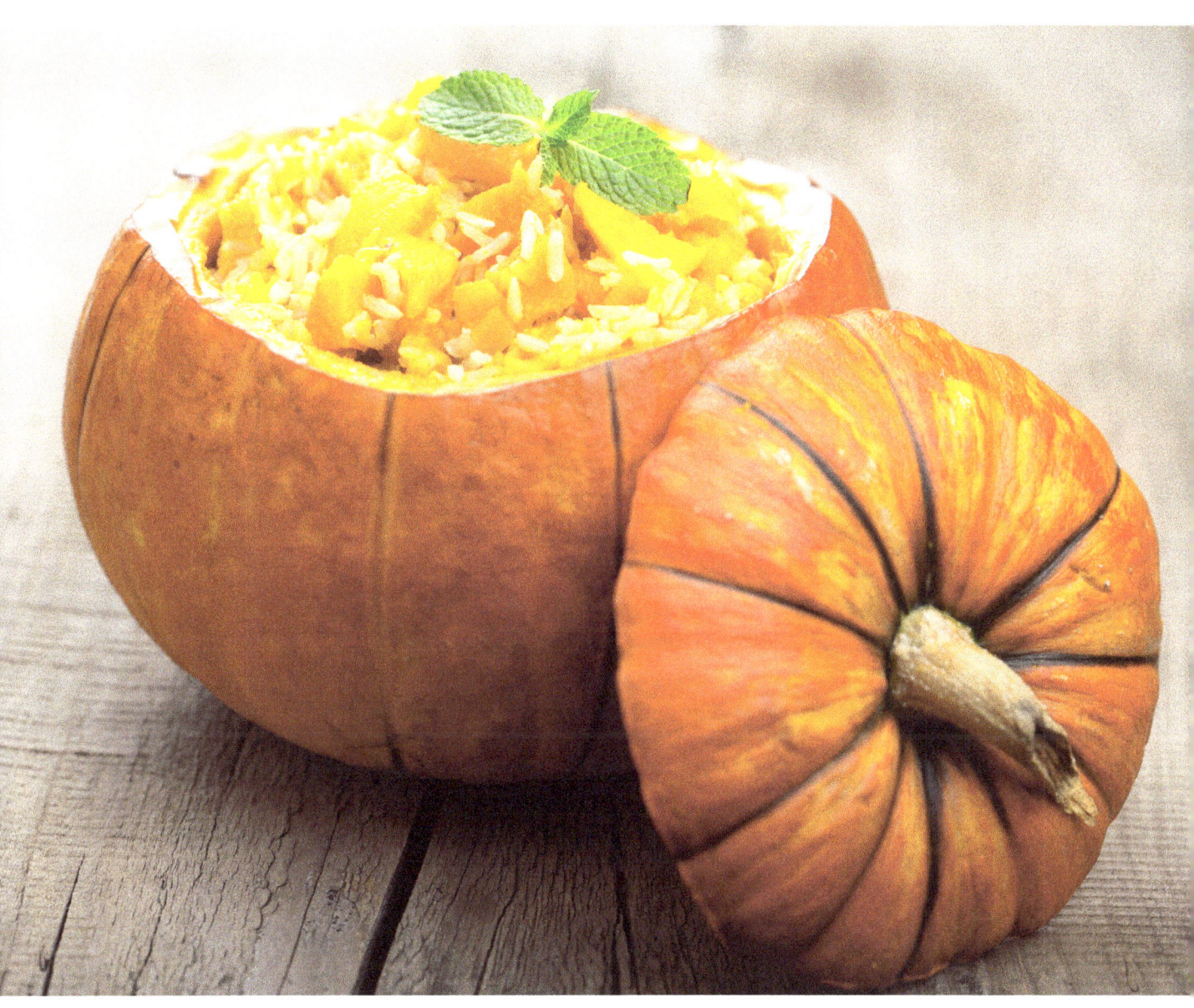

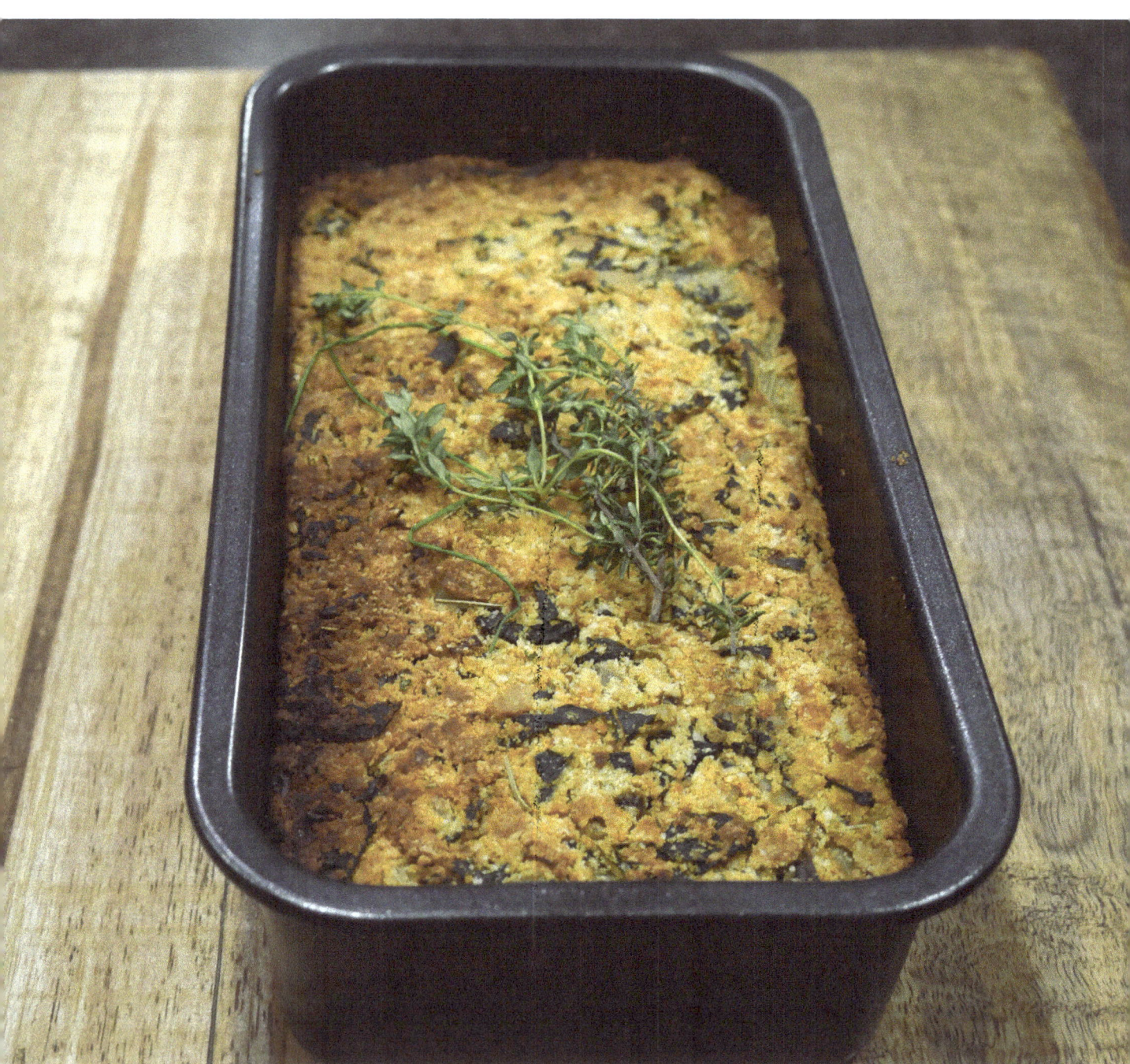

SPINACH AND ALMOND ROAST

Who doesn't love a roast dinner? This one is delicious, paired with your traditional roast vegetables and of course some gravy, this recipe is up there as one of the best. Enjoy.

PREPARATION TIME
40 MINUTES

COOKING TIME
30 MINUTES

SERVES
6

INGREDIENTS:

400gm spinach
1 large stick of celery
30ml garlic infused olive oil
240gm almond meal
200gm fresh wholewheat GF breadcrumbs
30gm tomato paste
15ml tamari
1gm dried marjoram
1gm mixed herbs
½ bunch fresh parsley, finely chopped
Sea salt and pepper to taste

METHOD:

1. Preheat oven 180°C.
2. Wash, chop and steam spinach until just tender.
3. Place spinach in colander and set aside to drain and cool.
4. Finely dice the celery.
5. Heat the oil in a fry pan, add the celery and cook until soft.
6. In a large bowl, add almond meal, breadcrumbs, mixed herbs, marjoram, parsley, salt and pepper mix together.
7. In a separate bowl, add spinach, tomato paste, tamari and celery. Blend.
8. Add spinach mix to dry mix. Mix together thoroughly and press into a greased loaf pan (or baking dish). Bake for ½ hour.

I find using fresh breadcrumbs works best for this recipe.

TOFU SPICED COUSCOUS

This dish is simple and can be eaten as a side or a main meal. Leftovers can be taken for work lunches the next day or a great salad at a BBQ (vegan of course ha!)

PREPARATION TIME
40 MINUTES

COOKING TIME
20 MINUTES

SERVES
8

INGREDIENTS:

600gm firm tofu – cut into 2cm cubes
60ml ricebran oil
black pepper
1 stick celery – finely diced
3gm ground turmeric
2gm ground ginger
225gm GF/low FODMAP couscous
375ml low FODMAP vegetable stock
100gm baby spinach leaves
75gm macadamias
½ avocado – diced
250gm punnet of cherry tomatoes – cut into quarters
30ml lemon juice
Lemon wedges for serving…

METHOD:

1. Toss tofu in 30ml of oil, season with salt and pepper.
2. Heat a large non-stick fry pan over high heat. Add tofu and cook turning occasionally until brown and cooked. Takes approx. 15 minutes. Remove from pan, cover and keep warm.
3. Heat 20ml oil in the same pan, add celery, cooking until just browning. Add turmeric and ginger. Cook, stirring for 30 seconds or until fragrant. Set aside.
4. Place couscous and stock in a saucepan. Cover with lid. Bring to boil. Once boiled, remove from heat.
5. Let couscous sit for 5 minutes. Fluff with fork to separate grains.
6. Toss avocado, tomato, spinach, nuts, lemon juice and remaining oil in a large bowl. Season with pepper.
7. Add tofu, celery and couscous and mix thoroughly but gently.
8. Serve with lemon wedges.

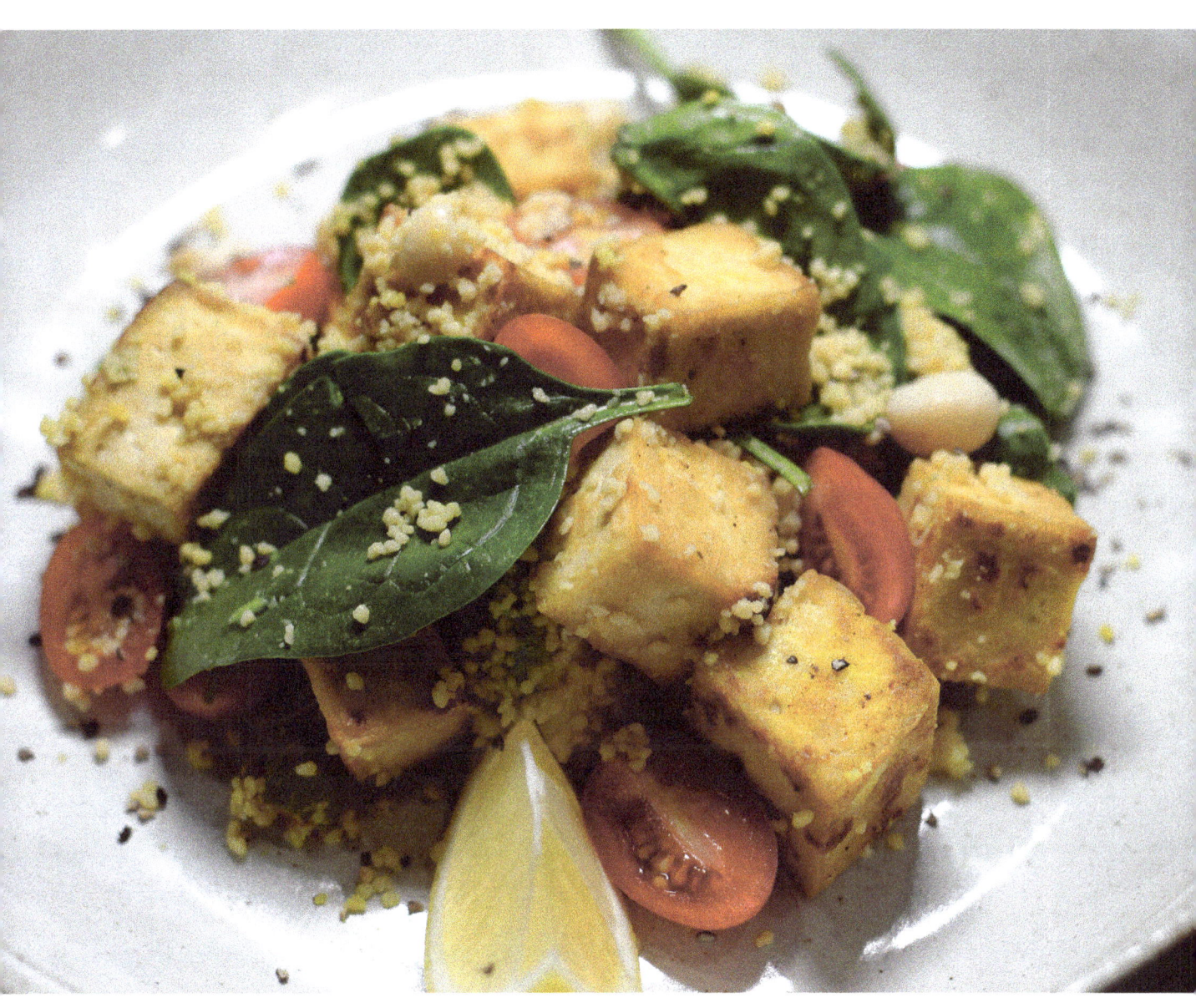

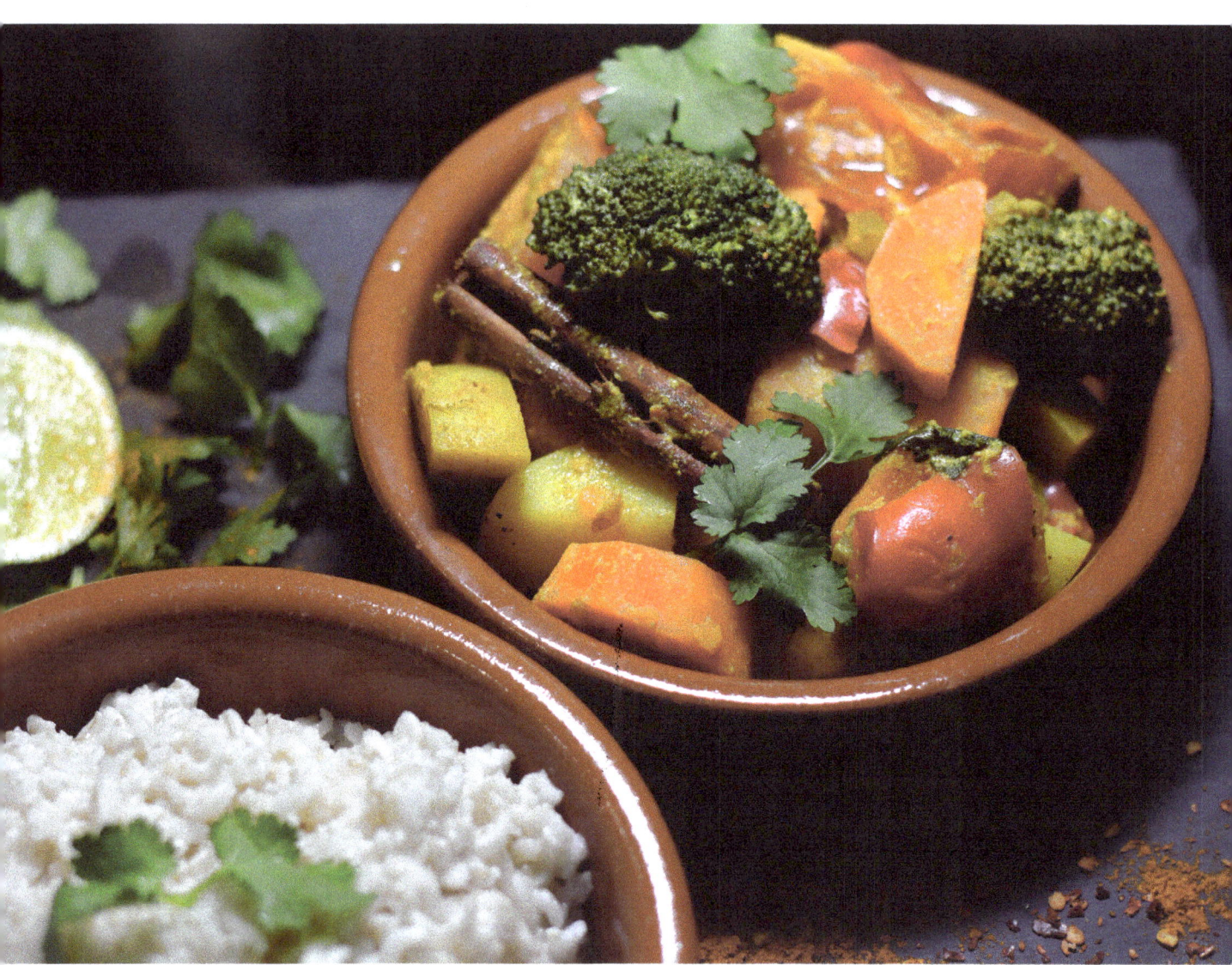

VEGETABLE CURRY WITH COCONUT RICE

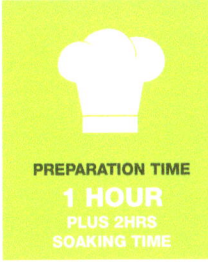
PREPARATION TIME
1 HOUR
PLUS 2HRS SOAKING TIME

COOKING TIME
30 MINUTES

SERVES
6

INGREDIENTS:

200gm brown rice
30ml garlic infused oil
(coconut oil works really well in this dish too)
2 cinnamon sticks
4 cloves
2 large celery sticks
1 can coconut milk
Himalayan sea salt – to taste
1kg mixed vegetables (pumpkin, carrots, beans, broccoli)
1 red capsicum
3 tomatoes
2gm turmeric
1gm powdered ginger
1gm ground coriander
4gm chili powder
5gm garam masala
250ml non-dairy milk

METHOD:

1. Cover rice with boiling water – leave to soak for 2 hours, drain.

2. Add drained rice to a saucepan and cover with coconut milk. Add enough water for the fluid to be approximately 2.5cm above the rice. Add a little salt, cover and bring to the boil. Reduce heat and simmer until tender – about 25 minutes.

3. Chop and steam vegetables until tender, drain and set aside.

4. Finely dice celery sticks and largely dice capsicum. Heat the garlic infused oil in a fry pan, fry celery and capsicum until just starting to soften, then add cinnamon and cloves and fry a further 4 minutes.

5. Slice the tomatoes into wedges.

6. Adding to the celery, stir in chopped tomatoes, turmeric, ginger, coriander, chilli powder, garam masala and a little salt to taste. Fry 3–4 minutes. Add cooked vegetables and non-dairy milk and cook until blended and hot.

Layer rice between 6 bowls and cover with the vegies.

Jodie Martin | **Chapter 5** Mains

RETRO BUBBLE AND SQUEAK PATTIES

This is a modern twist on a delicious old family favourite. Full of flavour, these patties take me back to my childhood. I hope they bring back special memories for you too.

PREPARATION TIME
45 MINUTES

COOKING TIME
10 MINUTES

SERVES
15 PATTIES

INGREDIENTS:

Garlic infused olive oil
1.5kg Potatoes washed and unpeeled.
1 cob corn
1 stick celery
1 Leek, green part only
3 Spring onions – green parts only
Bunch of kale
½ red capsicum
15gm savoury yeast flakes
60gm chia seeds
GF breadcrumbs – for rolling patties in
5gm Himalayan sea salt

METHOD:

1. Cut potatoes into 2cm square cubes, leaving the skin on.
2. Place in a large saucepan, cover with water, add 1 tsp Himalayan sea salt and bring to the boil.
3. Once boiled, reduce heat and let simmer until very well cooked through.
4. Place corn cob and water in a saucepan and bring to the boil. Once boiled, reduce heat and simmer approximately 5 minutes.
5. Once cooked, drain corn and allow to cool slightly. Once cooled, using an open flame on the stove top, char the corn so as areas start to go black.
6. Let cool and then cut the corn off close to the cob and place in a large mixing bowl.
7. Finely dice the celery and capsicum. Thinly slice the leek, spring onions and kale.
8. Heat oil in a fry pan, once hot add the chopped vegies and cook until just soft.
9. Add to corn in the mixing bowl.
10. When potatoes are cooked, drain and roughly mash. Add to the vegies, along with the savoury yeast flakes and chia seeds and mix until thoroughly blended. Season to taste.
11. When the mix is cool enough to handle, scoop out large spoonfuls and mould into a burger shape.
12. Roll in breadcrumbs and set aside on a tray lined with baking paper.
13. These are easiest rolled while the potato is still warm as it starts to go hard and 'set' as it cools.
14. Refrigerate until completely cold, then they can be put on the BBQ or browned off in a fry pan.

They are great as burgers or plated up with a side salad.

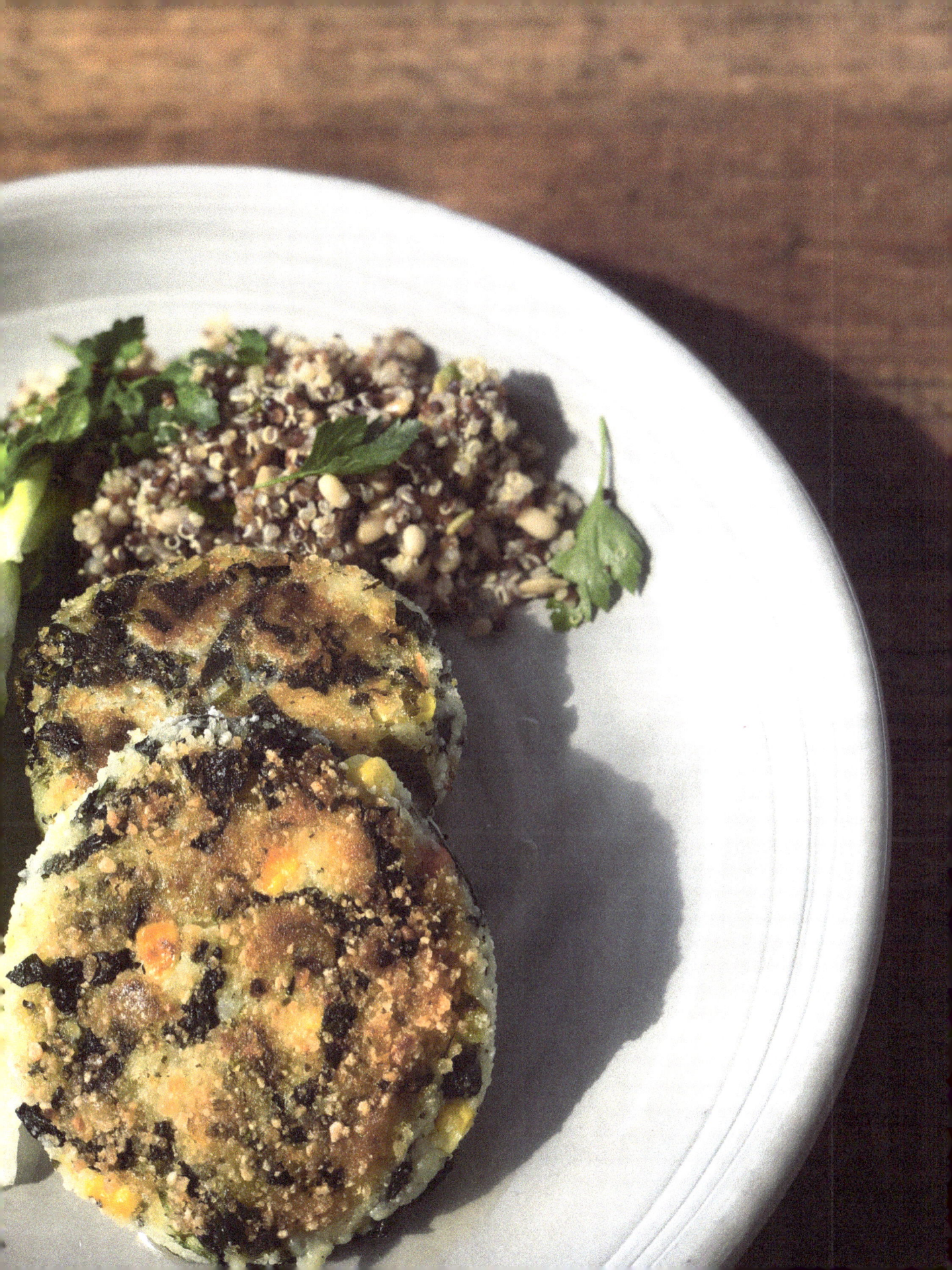

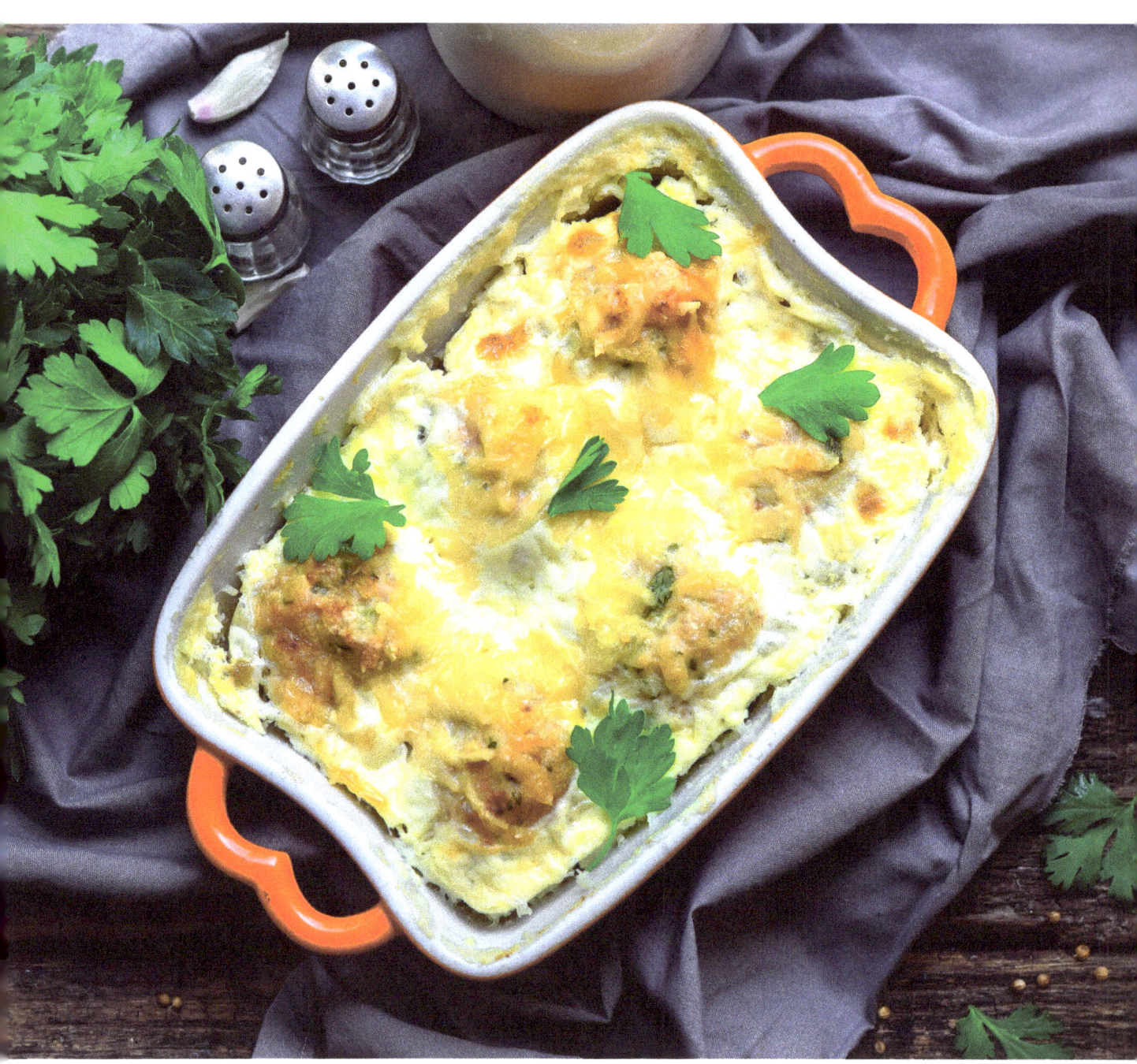

CHEESY VEGETABLE BAKE

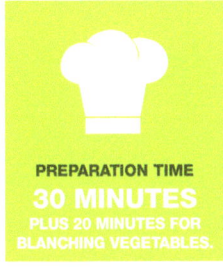
PREPARATION TIME
30 MINUTES
PLUS 20 MINUTES FOR BLANCHING VEGETABLES.

COOKING TIME
30 MINUTES

SERVES
8

INGREDIENTS:

6 cups of various vegies – sweet potato, broccoli, carrots, beans, squash, brussels sprouts, potatoes, parsnip, pumpkin etc.
1 serve of 'not' cheese sauce
Savoury yeast flakes for dusting (optional)

METHOD:

1. Preheat oven to 180°C.
2. Cut vegetables up into serving size pieces and steam until just soft.
3. Once softened through, drain all water from vegies and place in a casserole dish.
4. Prepare 1 serve of 'not' cheese sauce. (See page 142)
5. Pour over the prepared vegies until all the vegies are covered.
6. Sprinkle with savoury yeast flakes and bake in oven until it goes golden brown.

This can be served as a side or as a meal with a side salad. I always have it on its own and pile my plate high. My husband has nailed this and it is truly one of my favourite all time dinners we have.

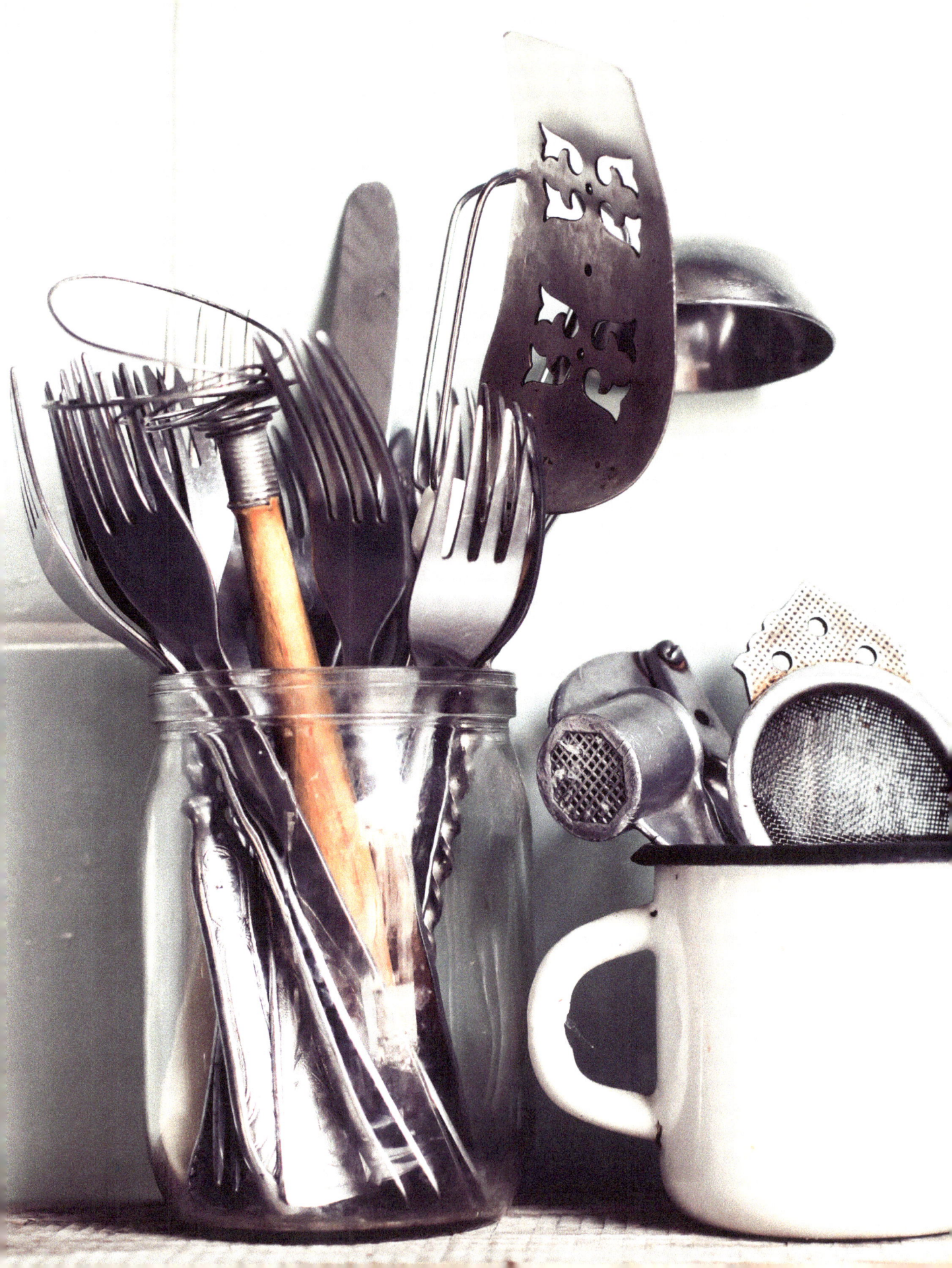

CHAPTER 6
Desserts

"The most damaging phrase in the language is: 'It's always been done that way'."
– Rear Admiral Grace Hopper

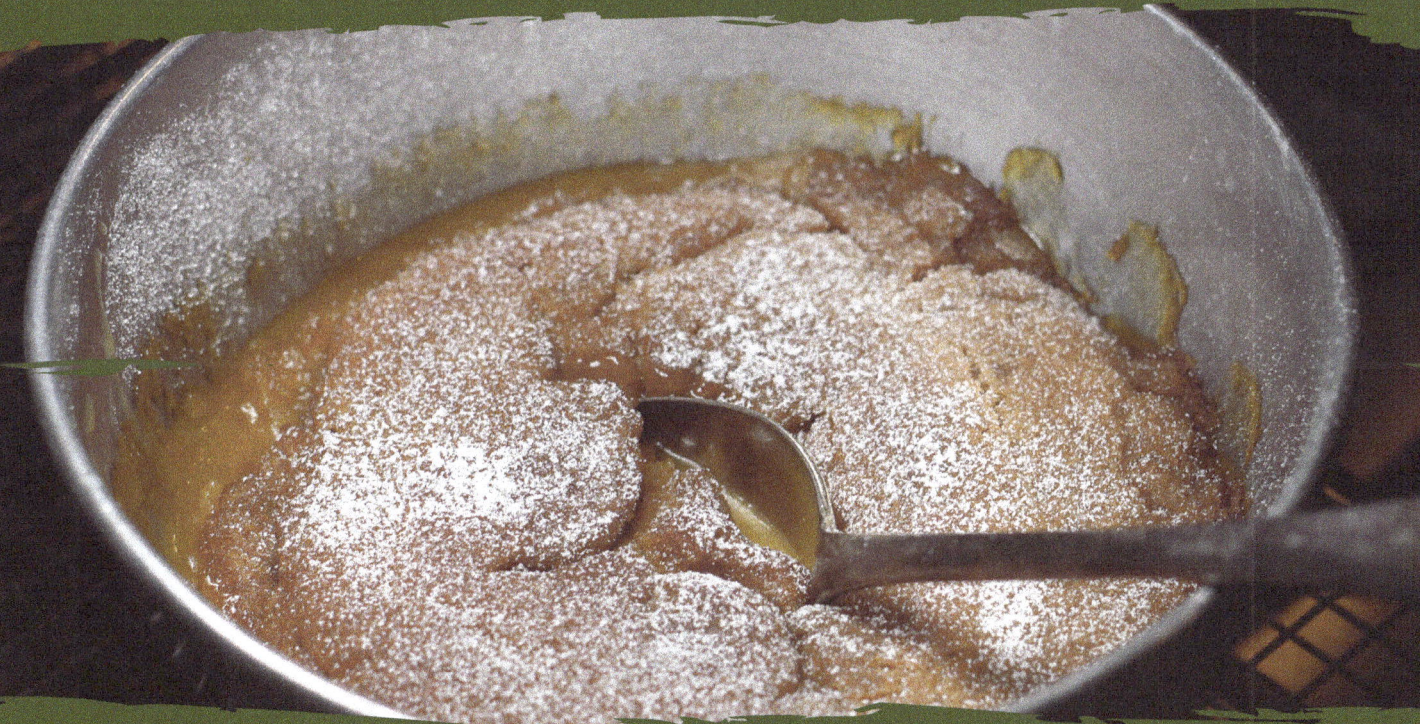

We all need balance in our life, right? So therein lies dessert… Enjoy these delicious dishes as my family does, showing a little restraint if possible.

Desserts are our naughty little treats. No! they are not super healthy but a great indulgence when eaten with controlled portion size -aargh, who am I kidding, you'll love these so much! You'll forget about control haha!

BAKED LEMON CHEESECAKE WITH RASPBERRY COULIS

This recipe sounds like it may be complex but actually it is really easy. Take this to any event and you will soon be the fan fav! Enjoy.

PREPARATION TIME
50 MINUTES

COOKING TIME
1 HOUR
PLUS 10 MINUTES

SERVES
12

INGREDIENTS:

BASE
160gm walnut meal
100gm GF plain flour
110gm sugar
100gm vegan butter – melted

FILLING
500gm vegan cream cheese
250gm soft tofu
210gm white sugar
Juice of 1 lemon
5ml vanilla essence

RASPBERRY COULIS
1 lemon
1 orange
500gm frozen raspberries
60gm sugar

METHOD:

1. Preheat oven to 180°C.
2. Line an 8inch spring form tin with baking paper and spray with oil any showing tin.
3. Place all ingredients for the base in a bowl and blend thoroughly.
4. Pour into the prepared tin, press into base and up the sides of the tin. Set aside.

For the filling:

5. Place all ingredients in a blender and blend until smooth and creamy.
6. Pour into biscuit base.

Bake 1 hour.

METHOD:

1. Juice the lemon and orange and place juice in a small saucepan.
2. Add raspberries and sugar and stir over low heat until the sugar dissolves.
3. Bring to the boil, then simmer until the mix starts to thicken and continue until desired thickness.
4. Mixture will thicken on standing.
5. When cheesecake has cooled, cut into slices and serve with the coulis.

www.SoulpodFoods.com.au

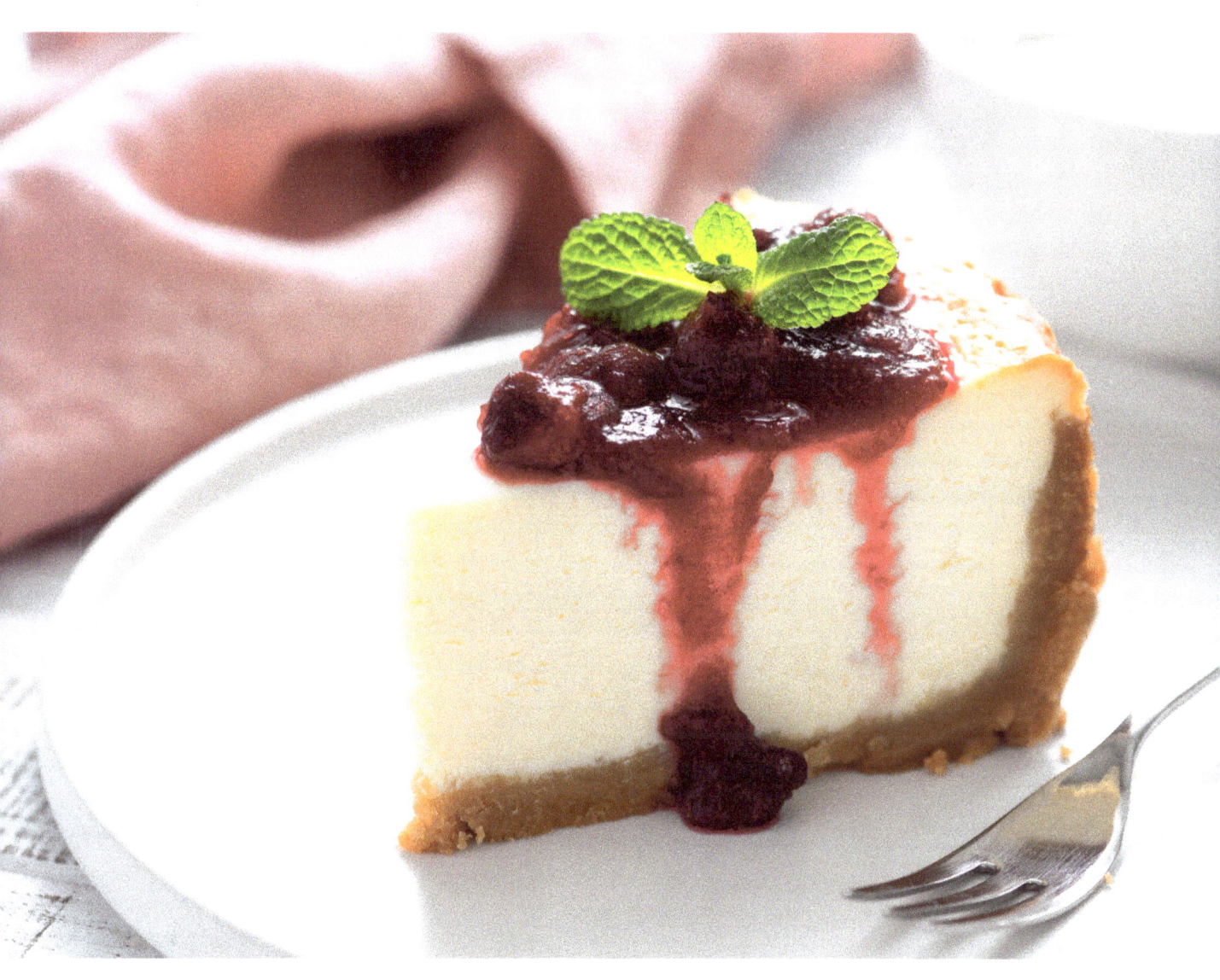

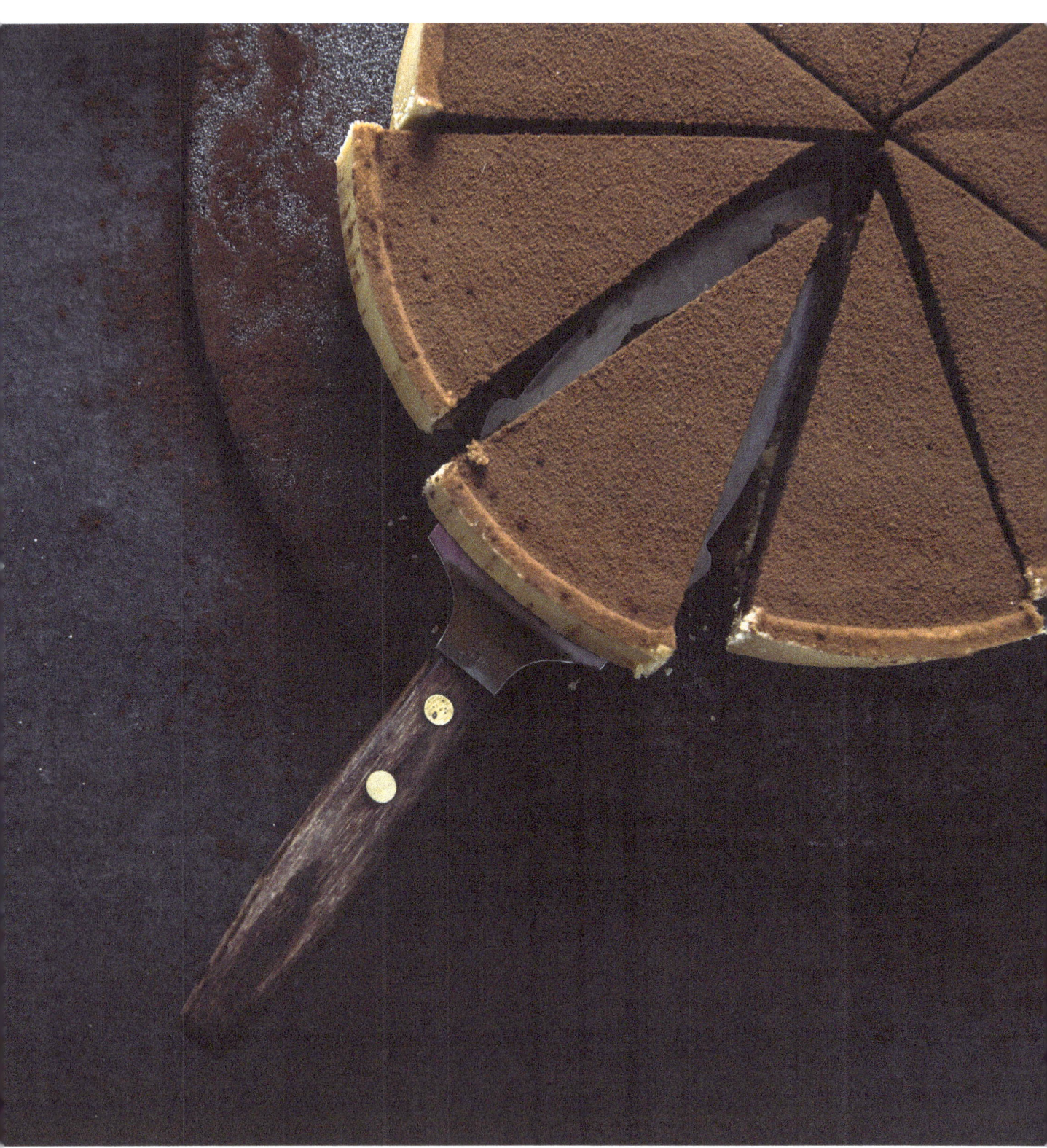

CHOCOLATE TORTE

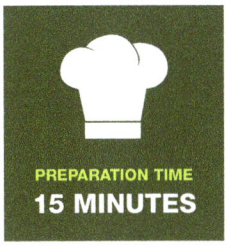
PREPARATION TIME
15 MINUTES

COOKING TIME
25 MINUTES
TOTAL

SERVES
8

INGREDIENTS:

310ml boiling water
5gm instant coffee
260gm bittersweet melting chocolate
2gm agar agar
5ml vanilla extract
2gm salt
Cacao for dusting
1.5 GF sweet shortcrust pastry sheets

METHOD:

1. Preheat oven to 180°C.
2. Thaw pastry sheet and line a greased pie dish. Poke with a fork creating small holes over the pastry. Cover with baking paper and top with baking beads.
3. Place in oven and blind bake until golden brown.
4. Place chocolate into a bowl.
5. Place coffee, agar agar and water into a saucepan, bring to the boil whisking constantly.
6. Once boiled, pour over the chocolate and stir until melted and smooth.
7. Add remaining ingredients and pour into the cooled pie crust.
8. Refrigerate minimum 6 hours.
9. Just before serving lightly dust with cacao.

This is quite a rich dessert. Serving with strawberries, kiwi fruit or other berries and some cheeky coconut ice cream really helps it to balance, so delicious.

Try adding a few drops of peppermint extract for those choc minty lovers.

VANILLA SLICES

PREPARATION TIME
1 HOUR

COOKING TIME
30 MINUTES
PLUS OVERNIGHT SETTING TIME

SERVES
12

INGREDIENTS:

2 sheets GF puff pastry
45gm GF custard powder
120gm castor sugar
600ml non-dairy milk
1 vanilla pod
20gm agar agar
250ml thickened unsweetened soy cream
Icing sugar – for dusting

METHOD:

1. Preheat oven 200°C.
2. Place the pastry on 2 baking paper lined trays and prick pastry with a fork numerous times.
3. Place in oven and cook until golden brown, approx. 10–15 minutes.
4. Once cooked, remove from oven and allow to cool on a cake rack.
5. In a medium size saucepan, blend custard powder, sugar and agar agar with enough of the milk to make a smooth paste.
6. Remove the vanilla bean paste from the vanilla pod, and add both to the custard mix. Over a moderate heat, slowly add the remaining milk whisking constantly to ensure it remains lump free and doesn't catch on the bottom of the saucepan.
7. Once boiled, simmer for one minute, then remove the vanilla pod.
8. Take off the heat and while still in saucepan, cover the custard with plastic wrap and allow to cool.
9. Line a square cake tin with grease proof paper and place pastry sheet in, cutting to size if required.
10. Once custard has cooled, add the soy cream and blitz on high speed with a stick blender until well blended and nice and creamy.
11. Pour custard into the cake tin, on top of initial pastry sheet and gently press the remaining pastry sheet on top of custard. Pushing gently but firmly to ensure no air bubbles and to smooth the custard.
12. Place in fridge over night to allow the custard to set.
13. Remove from fridge, with a sharp knife cut into desired size pieces, dust with icing sugar and enjoy!

www.SoulpodFoods.com.au

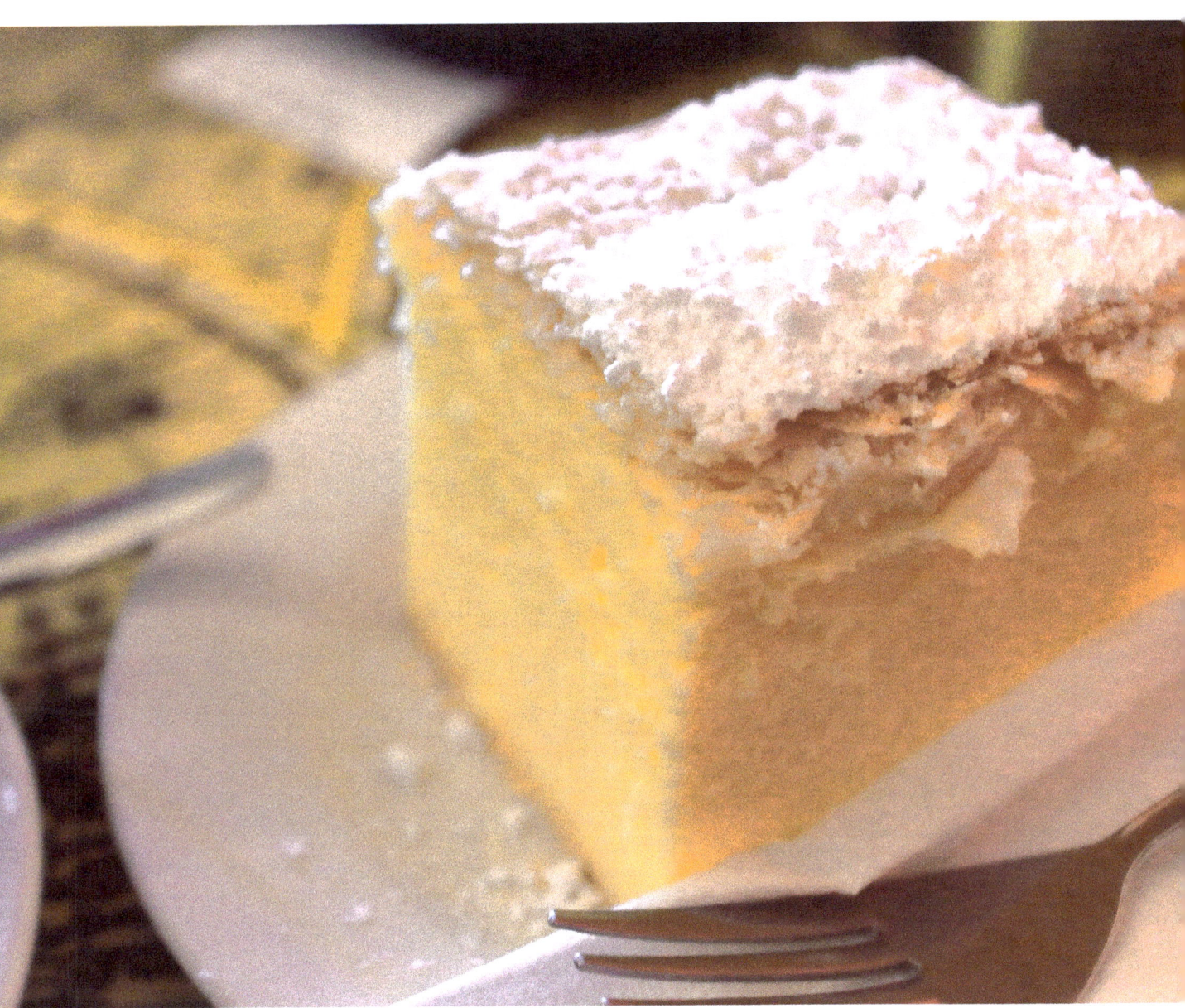

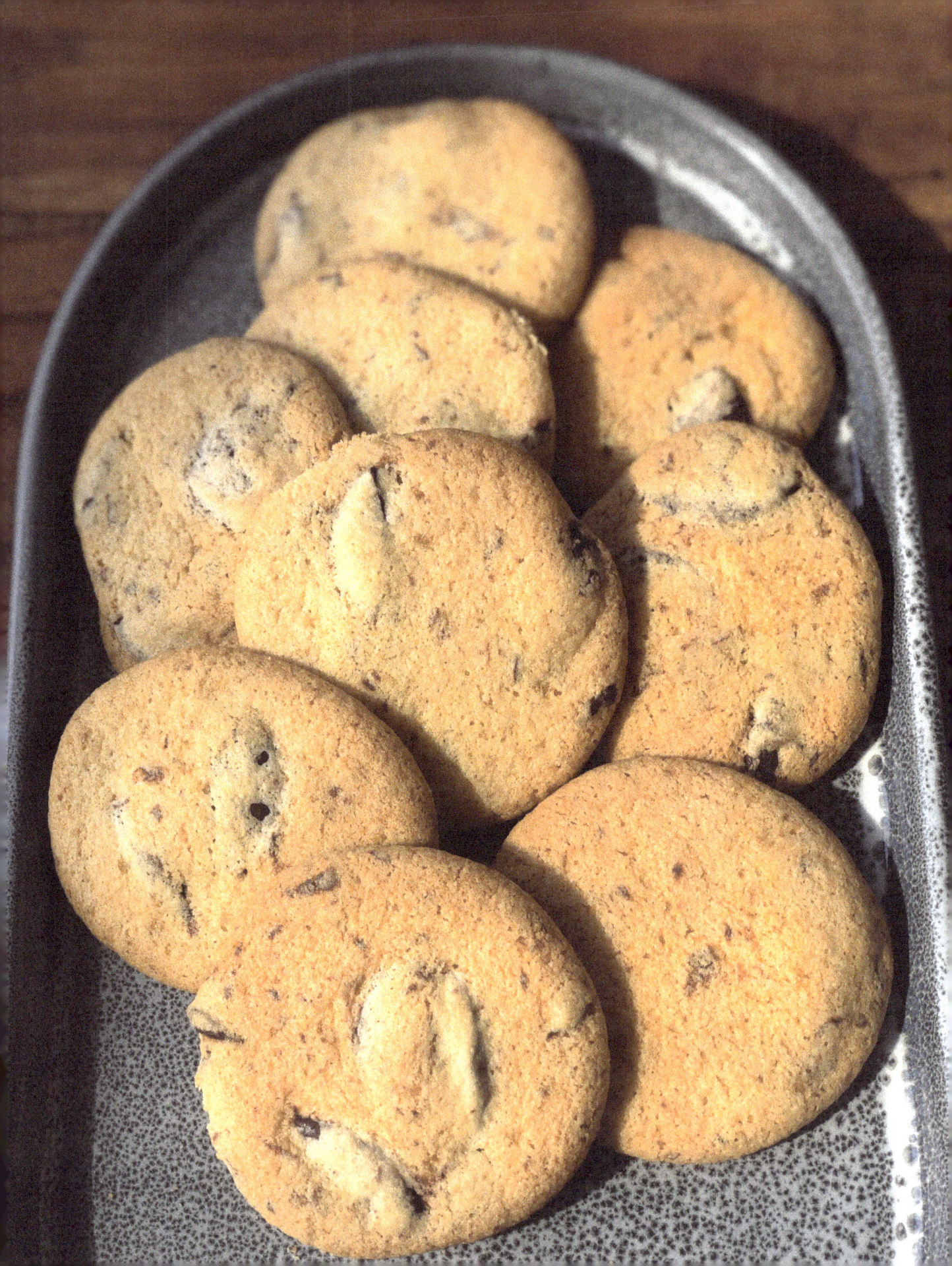

CHOCOLATE CHIP COOKIES

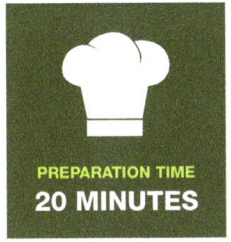
PREPARATION TIME
20 MINUTES

COOKING TIME
15 MINUTES

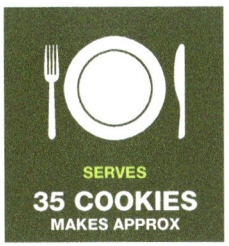
SERVES
35 COOKIES
MAKES APPROX

INGREDIENTS:

115gm vegan butter
100gm coconut sugar
170gm GF SR flour
100gm coconut condensed milk
150gm chocolate bits

METHOD:

1. Preheat oven to 190°C.
2. Place butter and sugar into a bowl and stir until well creamed.
3. Add flour and condensed milk and mix until well combined.
4. Add chocolate bits and mix through thoroughly.
5. Line an oven tray with baking paper.
6. With a teaspoon, scoop mix out and place on tray a good 5cm apart. Mixture will spread while cooking.
7. Place in oven and cook for 15 minutes. Slightly less for a chewier cookie.

These do make quite a large flat cookie. When placing on the tray, try and stick to the teaspoon size.

Jodie Martin | **Chapter 6** Desserts

MISO SALTED CARAMEL

PREPARATION TIME: 5 MINUTES
COOKING TIME: 15 MINUTES

INGREDIENTS:

210gm coconut sugar
1x 400gm can coconut cream
40gm GF shiro/white miso

METHOD:

1. Place all ingredients in a medium size saucepan.
2. Gently bring to the boil, stirring constantly to prevent catching.
3. Once boiled, reduce heat and let simmer for 6 minutes.
4. Stirring occasionally to prevent sticking.
5. Let cool slightly before pouring into a sterilised jar. Sauce will thicken slightly as it cools.
6. Store in fridge. Lasts approx 10 days.

This sauce is sticky and delicious. It can be used in smoothies, on pancakes, poured over sticky toffee pudding or enjoyed over non-dairy ice cream. My favourite is to dip fresh fruit into it – decadent.

www.SoulpodFoods.com.au

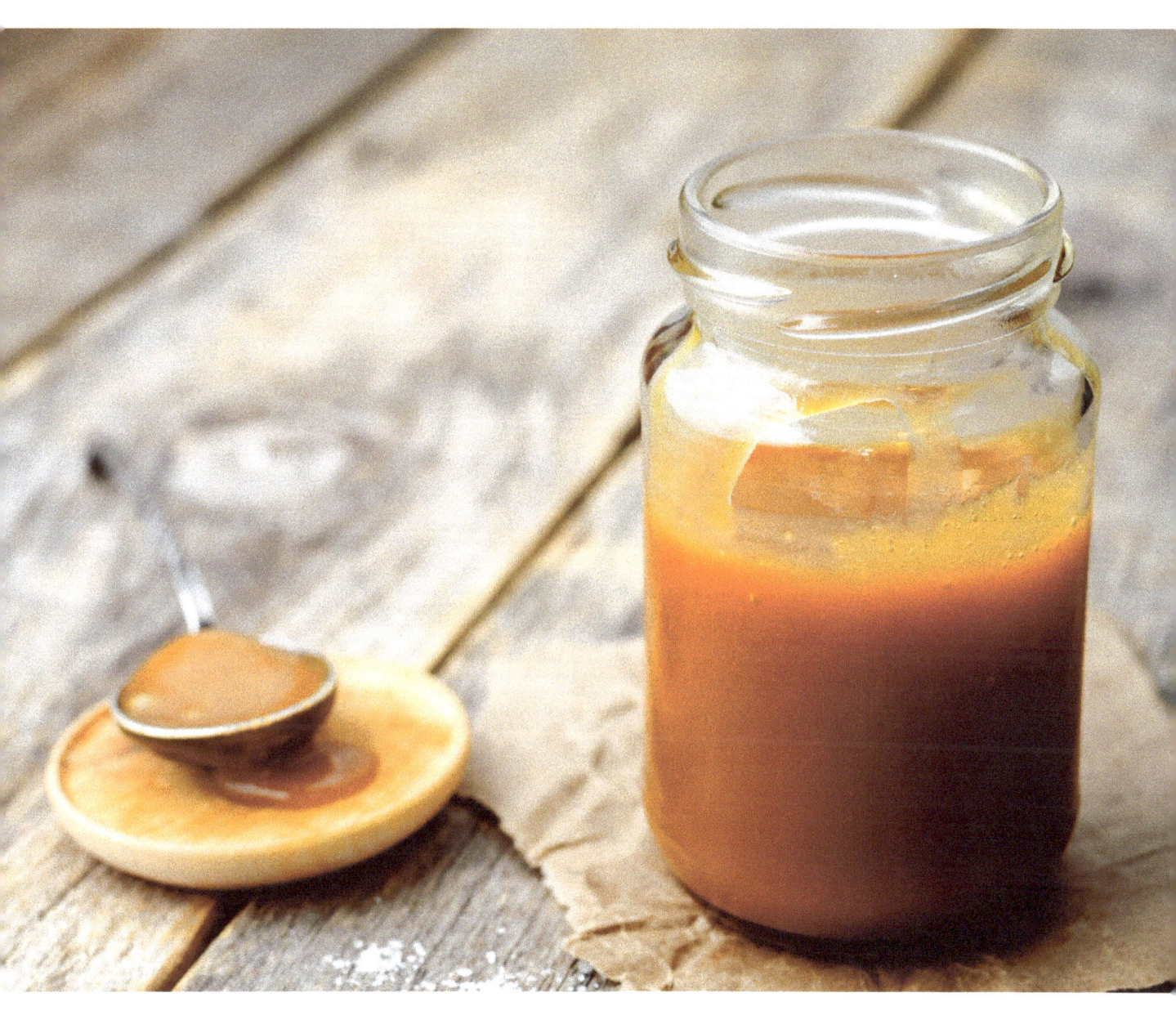

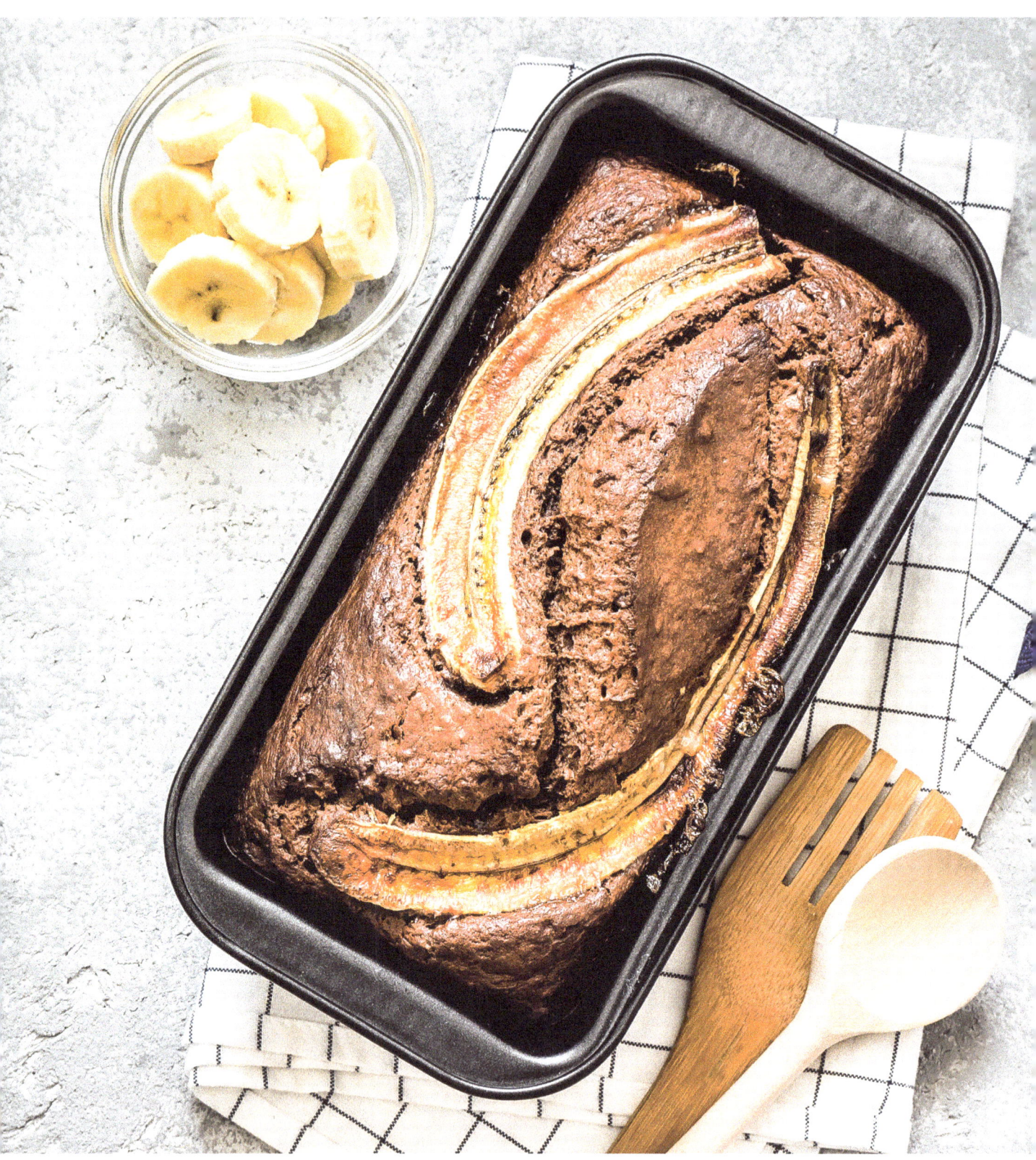

BANANA CHOCOLATE BREAD

PREPARATION TIME 30 MINUTES
COOKING TIME 50 MINUTES

INGREDIENTS:

Ingredients:
195gm GF SR flour
2gm Himalayan sea salt
100gm coconut sugar
65ml coconut oil, melted
4 bananas, mashed
5ml vanilla essence
200gm choc bits
Extra banana

METHOD:

1. Preheat oven 160°C.
2. Grease a standard loaf tin.
3. In a large bowl, combine sugar and oil. Whisk together.
4. Add the banana's, the vanilla, stirring until thoroughly mixed.
5. In a bowl, combine flour and salt. Mix together.
6. Add flour to the banana mix and stir until just wet.
7. Pour into prepared pan, place a banana sliced lengthways along top of mix and bake for 50 minutes or until a skewer comes out clean when tested.

BUTTERSCOTCH PUDDING

PREPARATION TIME
20 MINUTES

COOKING TIME
35 MINUTES

SERVES
6

INGREDIENTS:

145gm GF SR flour
100gm coconut sugar
2gm salt
60gm plant-based butter, melted
125ml non-dairy milk
60ml 100% maple syrup
30gm extra plant-based butter
375ml boiling water

METHOD:

1. Preheat oven 180°C.
2. In a large bowl place GF SR flour, sugar and salt. Mix through.
3. Add melted butter and the milk. Mix thoroughly.
4. Place in a greased deep dish.
5. In a small saucepan, combine the maple syrup, extra butter and hot water.
6. Stir over a low heat until the butter melts.
7. Pour over the pudding mixture.
8. Bake in oven 35 minutes. Pudding is cooked when skewer comes out clean when checked.
9. Serve with coconut ice cream.

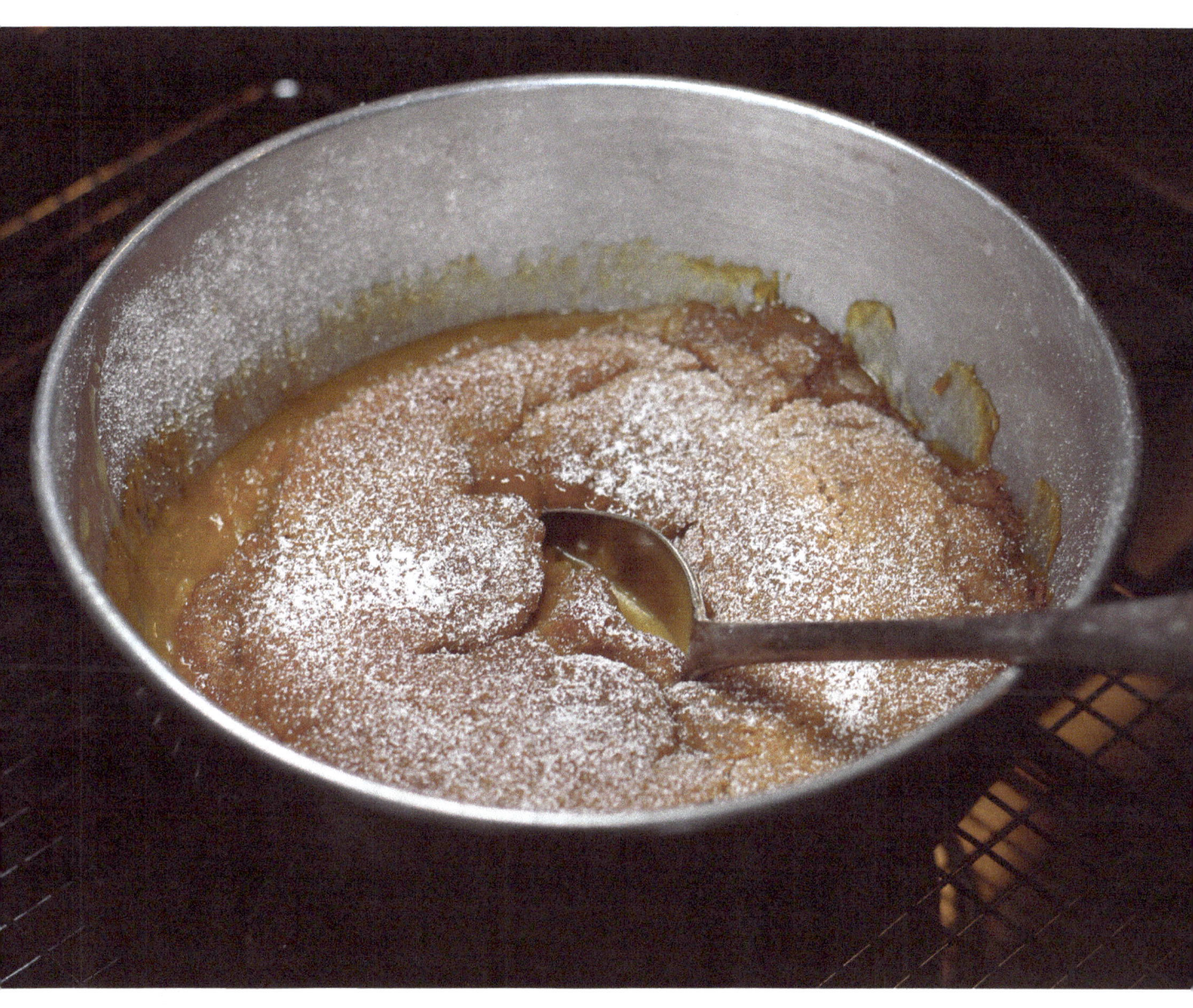

Jodie Martin | **Chapter 6** Desserts

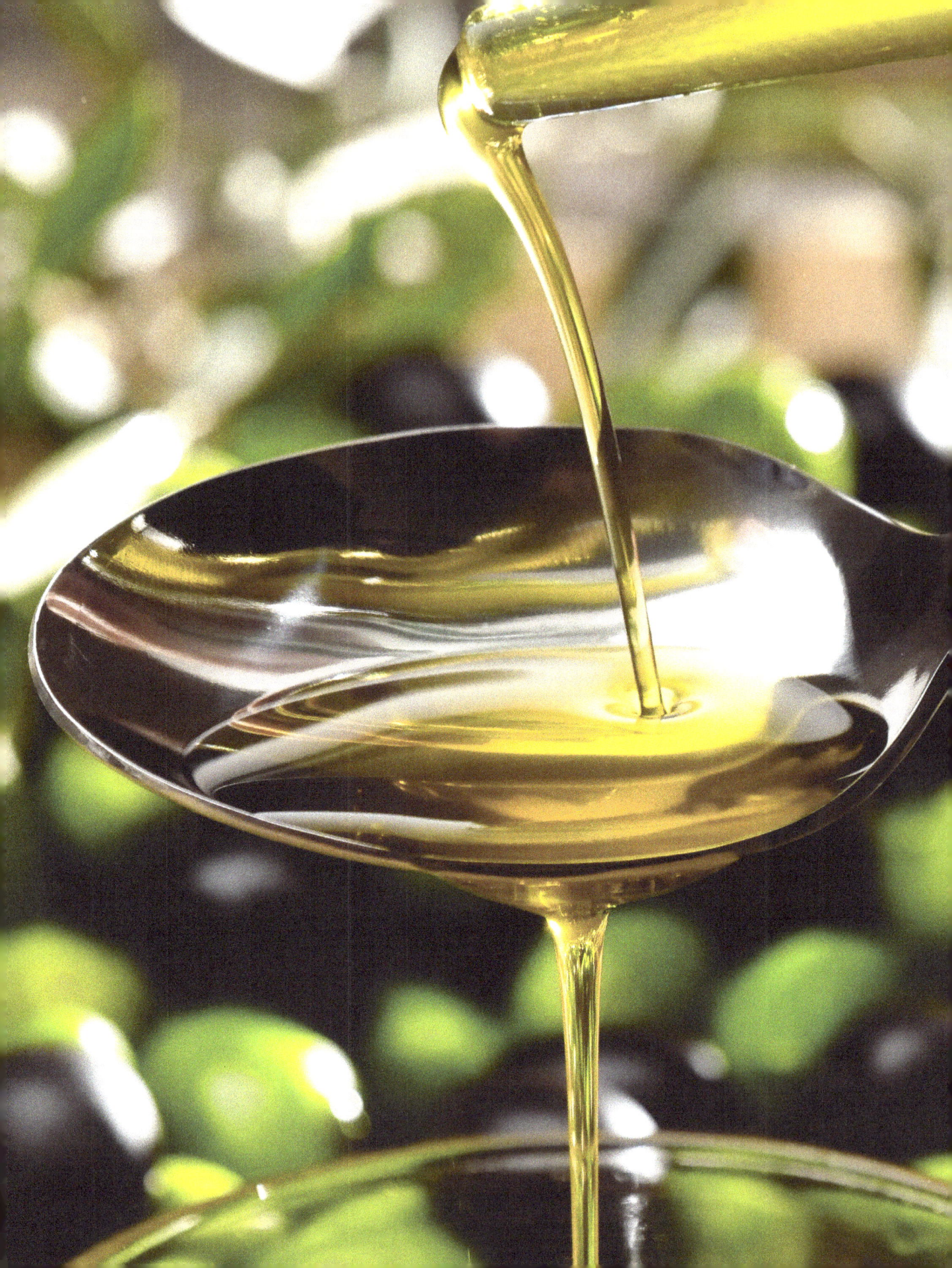

CHAPTER 7
Bits and Pieces

"Do unto others as you would have them do unto you."
– Bible MATTHEW 7:12

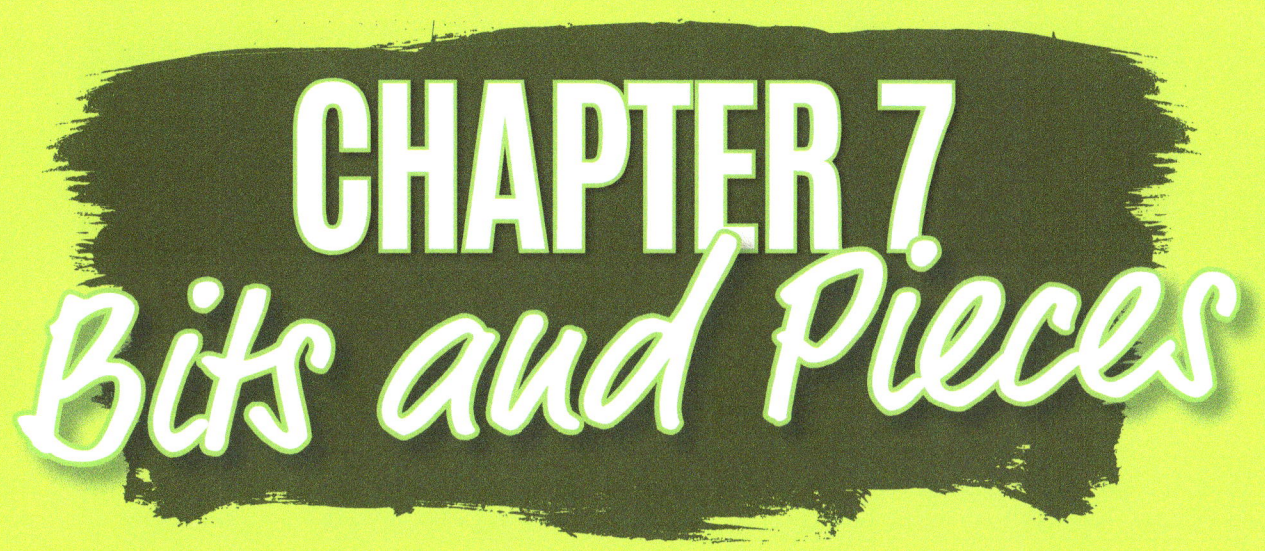

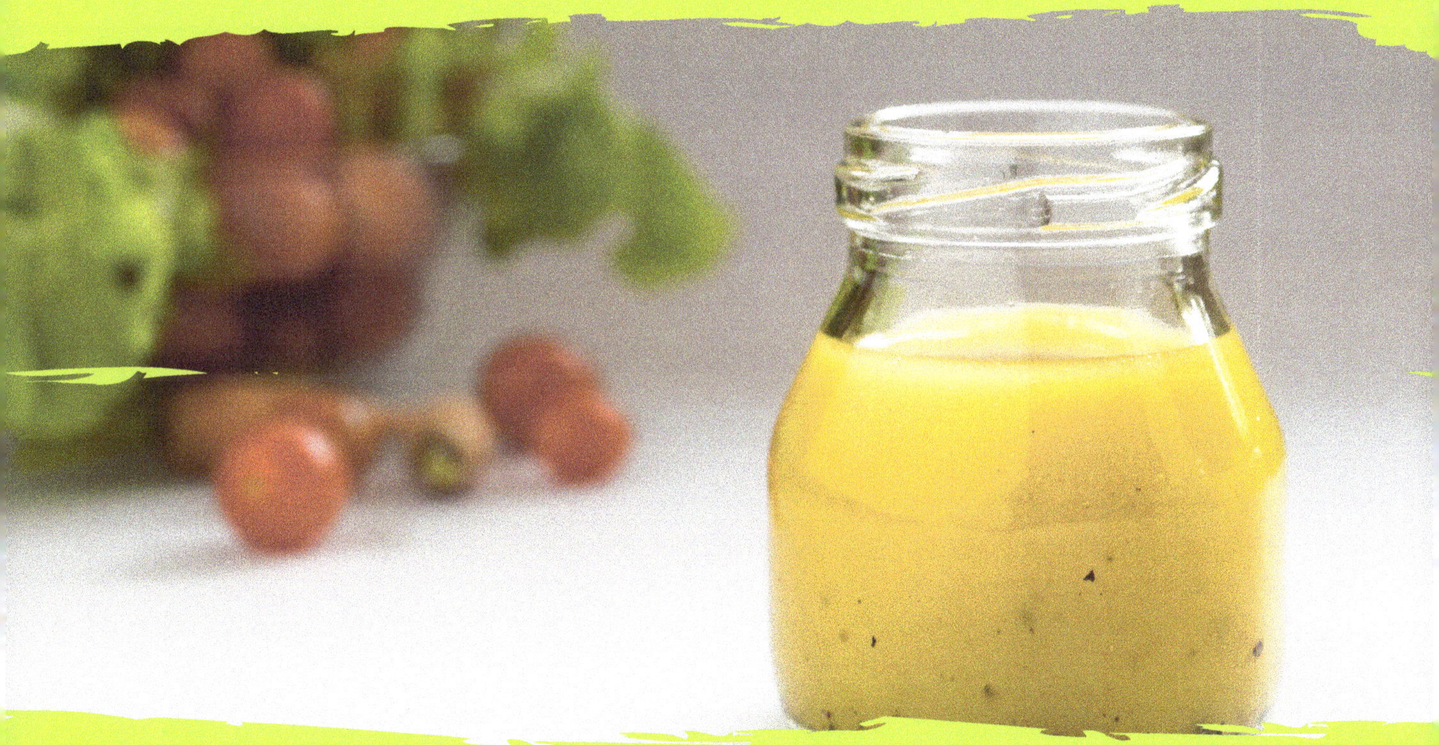

We can make the greatest of dishes but often it's the little added extras that can create heroes on the plate. The following are some little gems that are my family's favourites. Within these gems, are a load of vitamins and minerals that are added value to the dish. If we can up our nutrient content – then why wouldn't we?

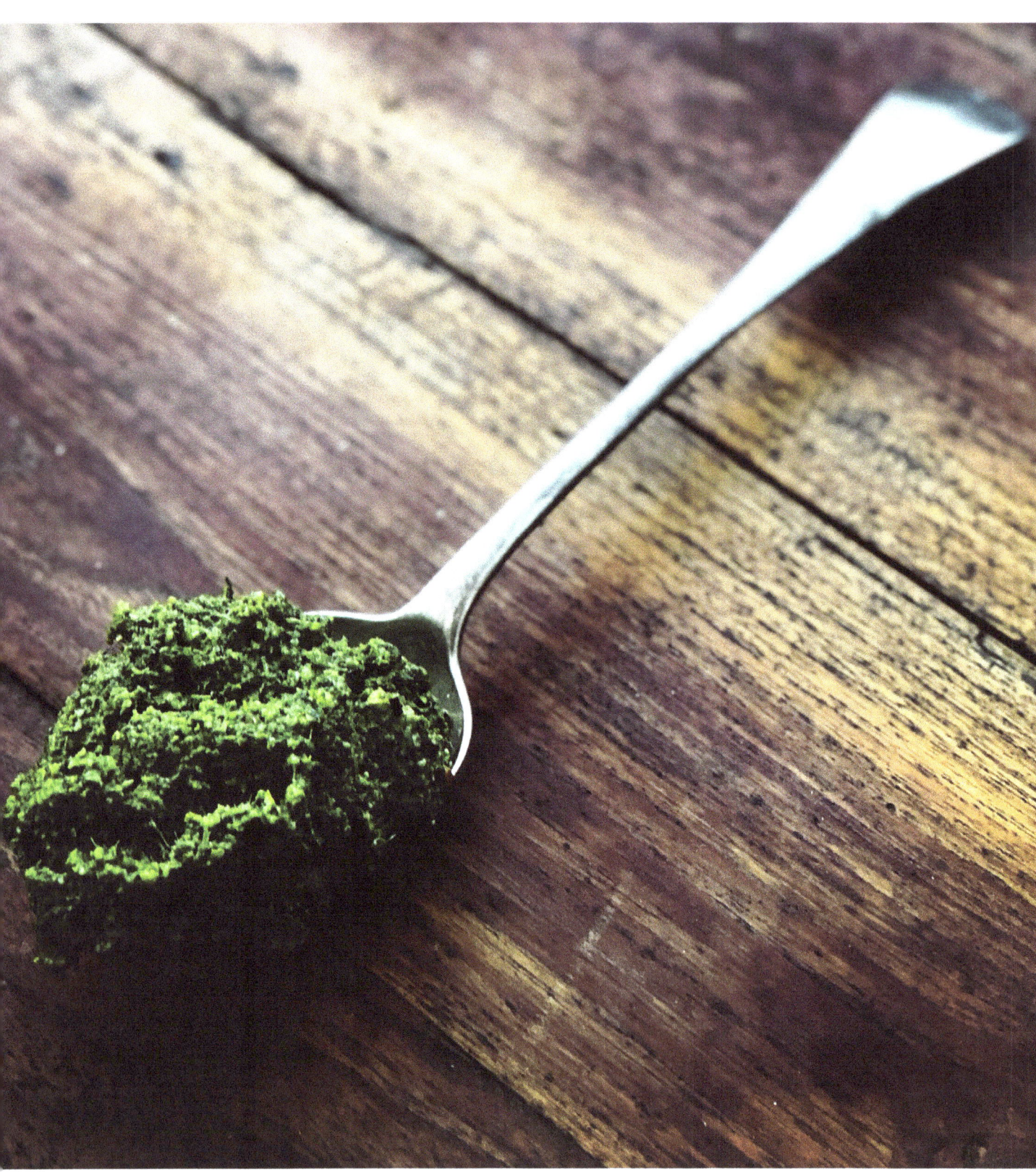

MACADAMIA NUT PESTO

PREPARATION TIME
10 MINUTES

COOKING TIME
5 MINUTES

INGREDIENTS:

100gms macadamia nuts
100gms pinenuts
40gm fresh basil
150ml garlic infused oil
6gm Himalayan sea salt
1gm cracked pepper
Savoury yeast flakes (optional)

METHOD:

1. In a dry non-stick fry pan, add nuts on a low heat and constantly stir until they start to brown, set aside.

2. Place all ingredients including the nuts into a blender and blitz until a thin paste or desired consistency.

This is delicious as a gnocchi pesto, inside arancini balls or a variety of different uses.

MACADAMIA FETA

PREPARATION TIME
OVERNIGHT + 15 MINUTES

COOKING TIME
4 HOURS IF DEHYDRATING

INGREDIENTS:

125gm raw macadamias, soaked overnight
100ml lemon juice
100ml water
5gm Himalayan sea salt
45ml garlic infused oil
1 probiotic (optional)

METHOD:

1. Place macadamias in a large bowl. Cover with water and set aside overnight.

2. Drain macadamias, place in a blender with the rest of the ingredients. Blend until creamy and smooth (may take 10 minutes)

3. Place in muslin cloth or nut bag, squeeze excess fluid out by twisting the cloth, forming a round ball.

4. Secure and place over a strainer in the fridge and let drain overnight.

5. You can use straight away or for a firmer cheese, dehydrate for minimum 4 hours.

6. Keep in fridge for 7–10 days.

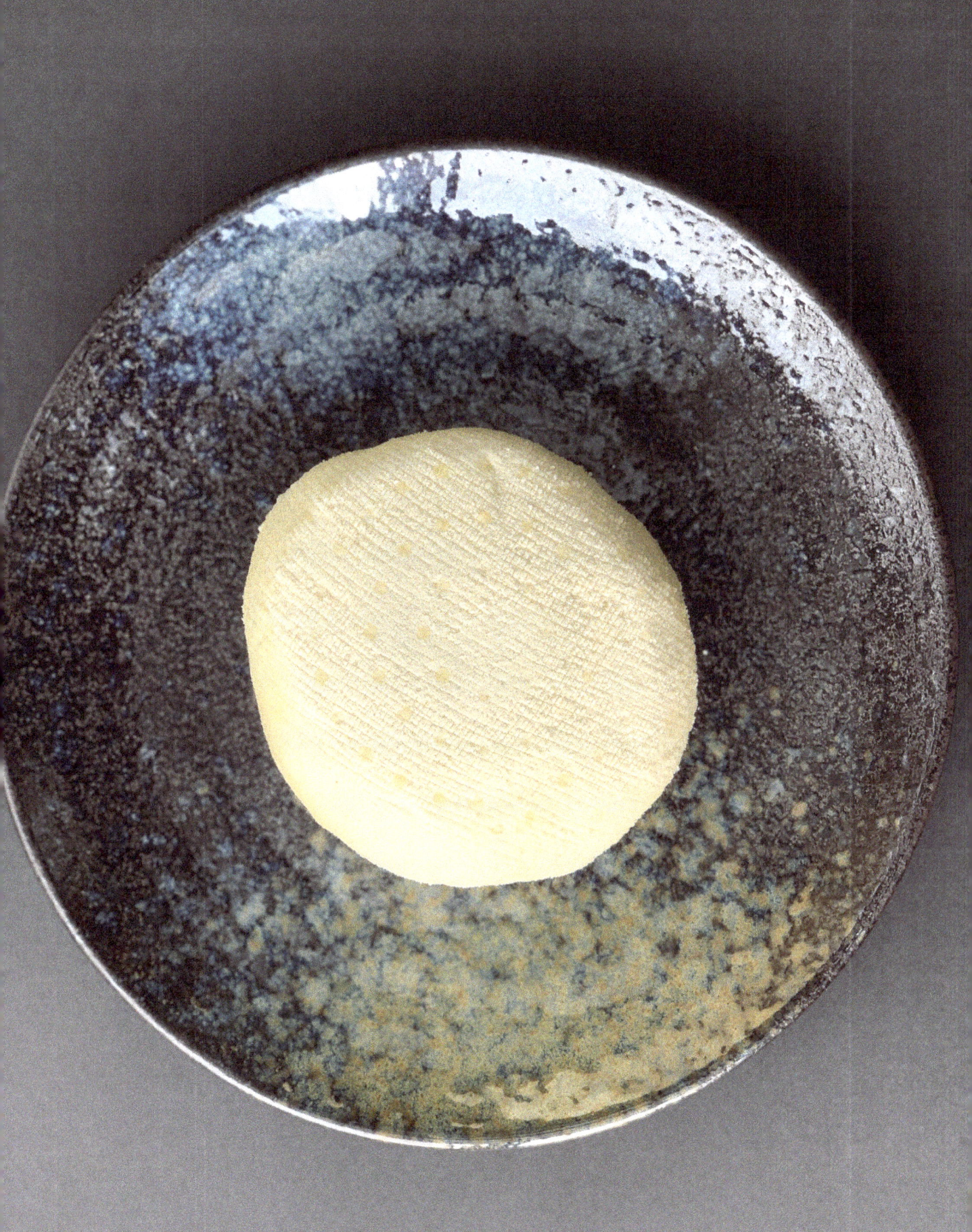

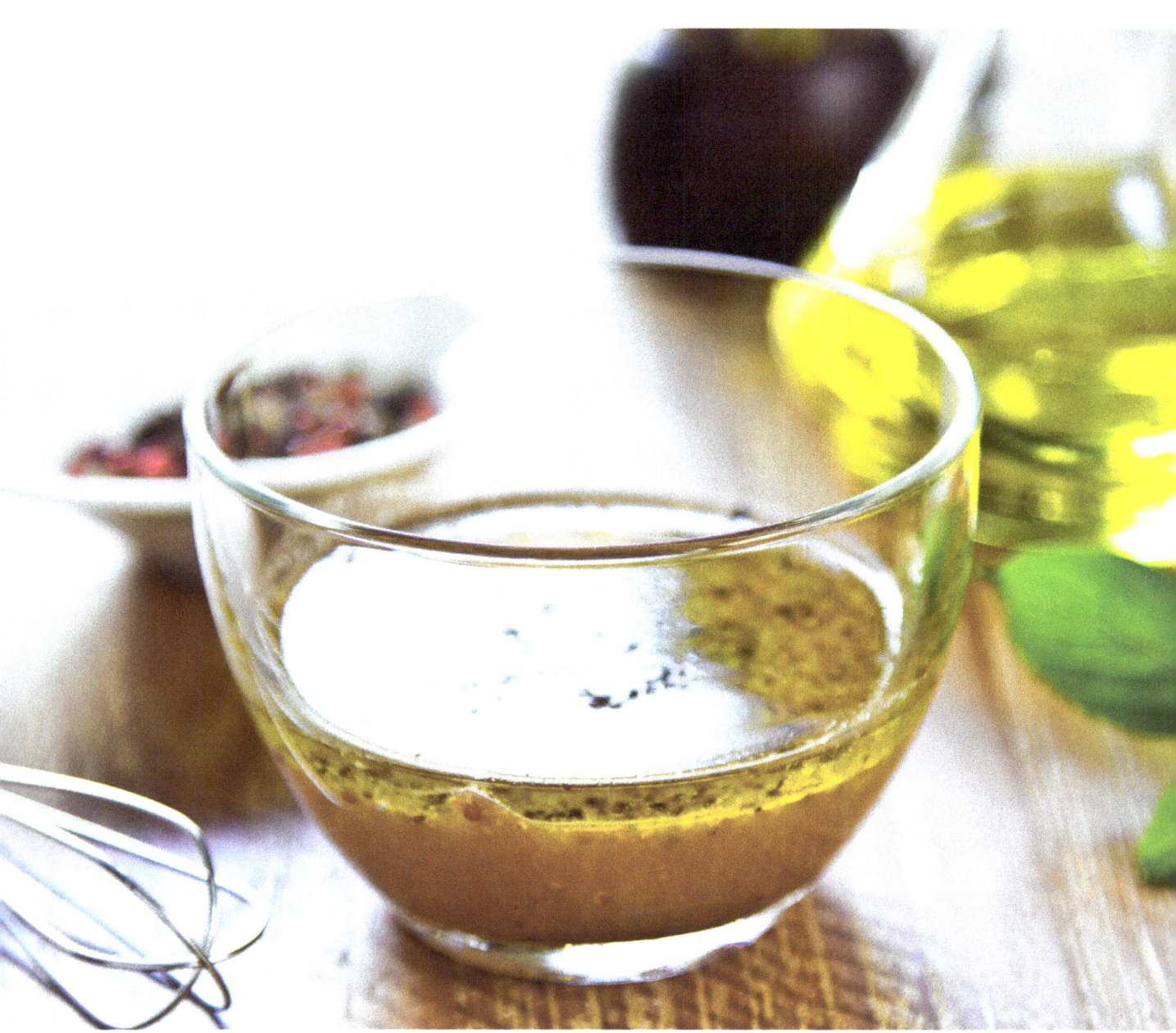

SALAD DRESSING

**PREPARATION TIME
10 MINUTES**

INGREDIENTS:

170ml oil – choose a good quality oil such as olive, macadamia, avocado or walnut
90ml white vinegar
3gm wet or 1gm dry mustard (not the hot variety)
Juice of ½ lemon
Salt and pepper to taste

METHOD:

Add all ingredients in a sealable container and shake until blended.

You can use this as a basic dressing or jooj it up with finely chopped thyme, rosemary, oregano, curry powder or whatever takes your fancy.

TZATZIKI

**PREPARATION TIME
30 MINUTES**

INGREDIENTS:

2 continental cucumbers (700 grams, or 3 Lebanese cucumbers)
5gm sea salt
500gm unsweetened coconut yogurt
50ml garlic infused oil
45ml lemon juice
1.5gm fresh mint
1gm fresh dill
Black pepper to taste

METHOD:

1. Cut cucumbers in half lengthwise, deseed with a teaspoon.

2. Grate or finely chop cucumbers. Add a teaspoon of salt, mix through and let stand for about 10 or 15 minutes in a sieve over a bowl.

3. Put cucumbers in a napkin, towel or cheesecloth and drain them and squeeze as much liquid out as you can.

4. Place the yogurt in a bowl, add the cucumbers, the garlic oil, lemon juice, black pepper to taste, mint and dill. You can add more salt if you want.

5. Stir and let stand for at least three or four hours in the fridge before serving to allow flavours to develop.

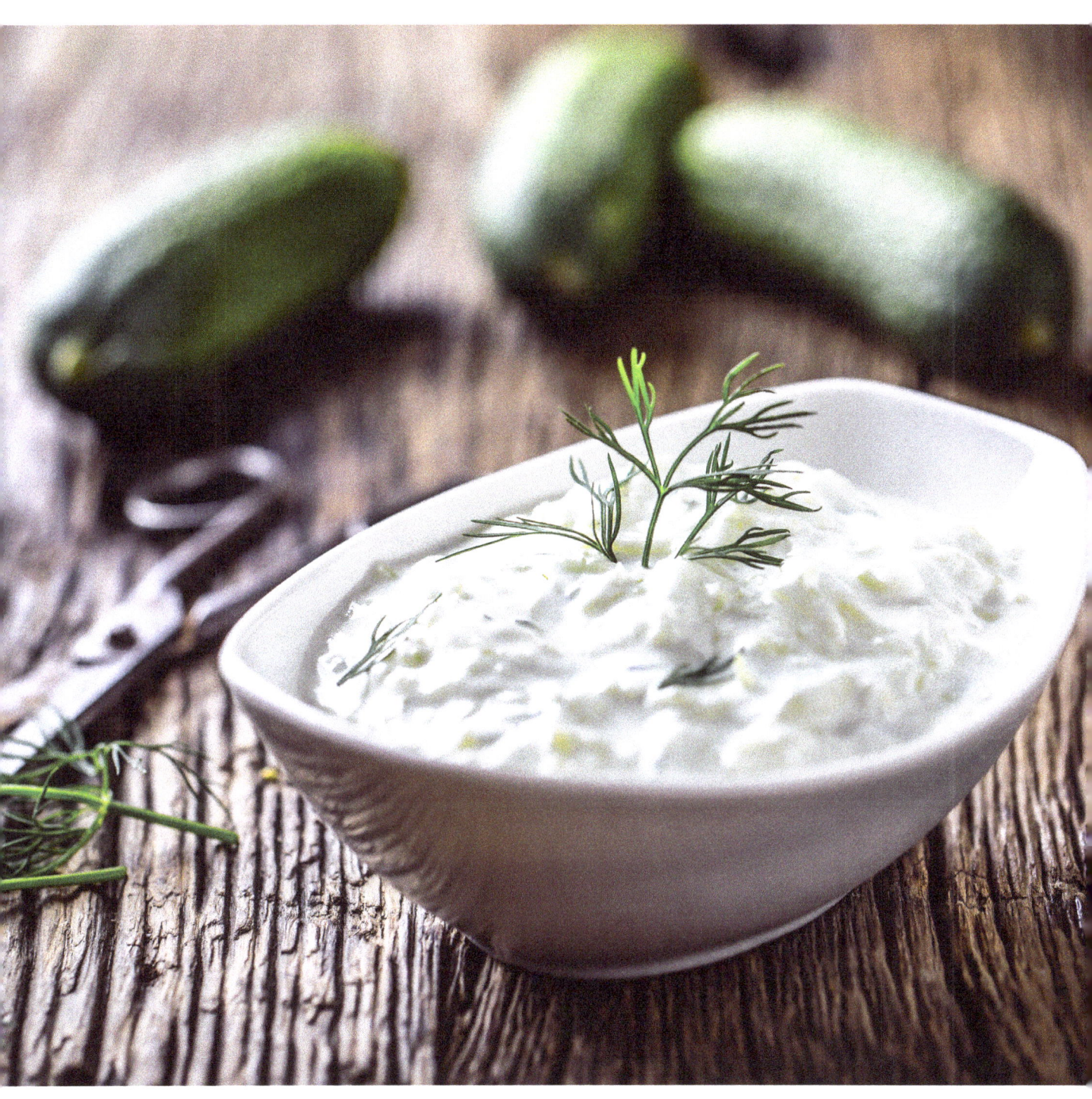

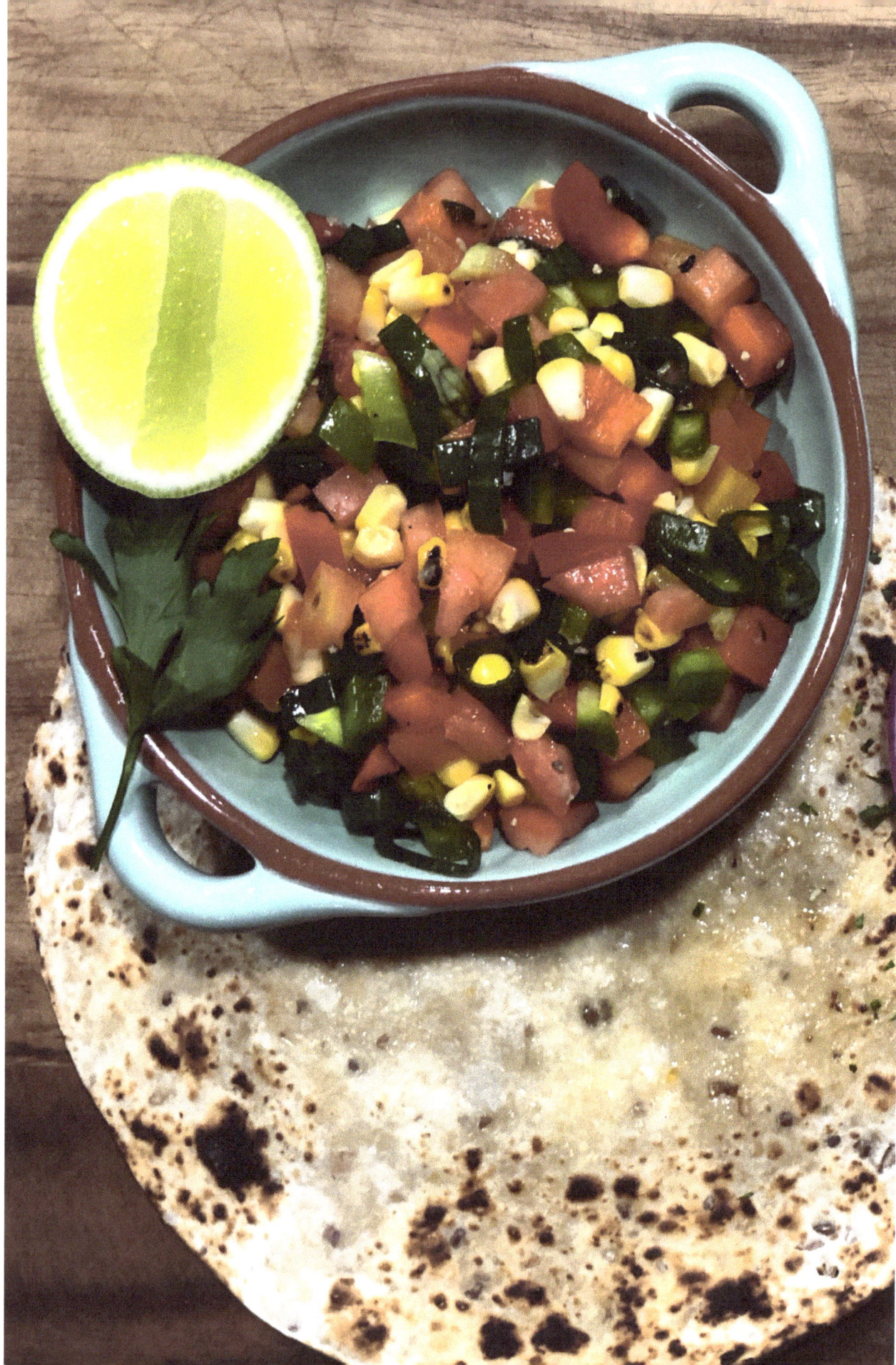

LIME SALSA

**PREPARATION TIME
20 MINUTES**

INGREDIENTS:

1 small red capsicum – finely chopped
1 small green capsicum – finely chopped
3 spring onion – green parts only
2 tomatoes- deseeded and finely chopped
1 corncob
½ lime
salt and pepper to taste.
5gm brown sugar (optional)

METHOD:

1. Boil corncob in a saucepan of salty water for about 5 minutes.
2. Let cool and dry off.
3. Once cool, chargrill on BBQ or on open flame on stove, until it starts to turn black.
4. Cut the corn off the cob and place in a bowl.
5. Dice capsicums, add to corn.
6. Deseed tomato and dice, place in bowl with corn and capsicum.
7. Finely slice the spring onions, add to the bowl.
8. Stir until thoroughly blended.
9. Squeeze juice of the lime over the salsa.
10. Add salt and pepper to taste.

NOT CHEESE SAUCE

PREPARATION TIME
10 MINUTES

COOKING TIME
20 MINUTES

INGREDIENTS:

600 ml soymilk
10gm GF plain flour
20gm vegan margarine
170gm savoury yeast flakes
salt and pepper to taste

METHOD:

1. In a saucepan, make a paste with the flour and margarine.
2. Over a moderate flame, slowly add the milk while constantly whisking the mix until smooth.
3. Continue whisking, increasing flame to high and continue stirring until mixture thickens.
4. Once thick, add the SYF, salt and pepper to taste and continue stirring until mixed thoroughly.

www.SoulpodFoods.com.au

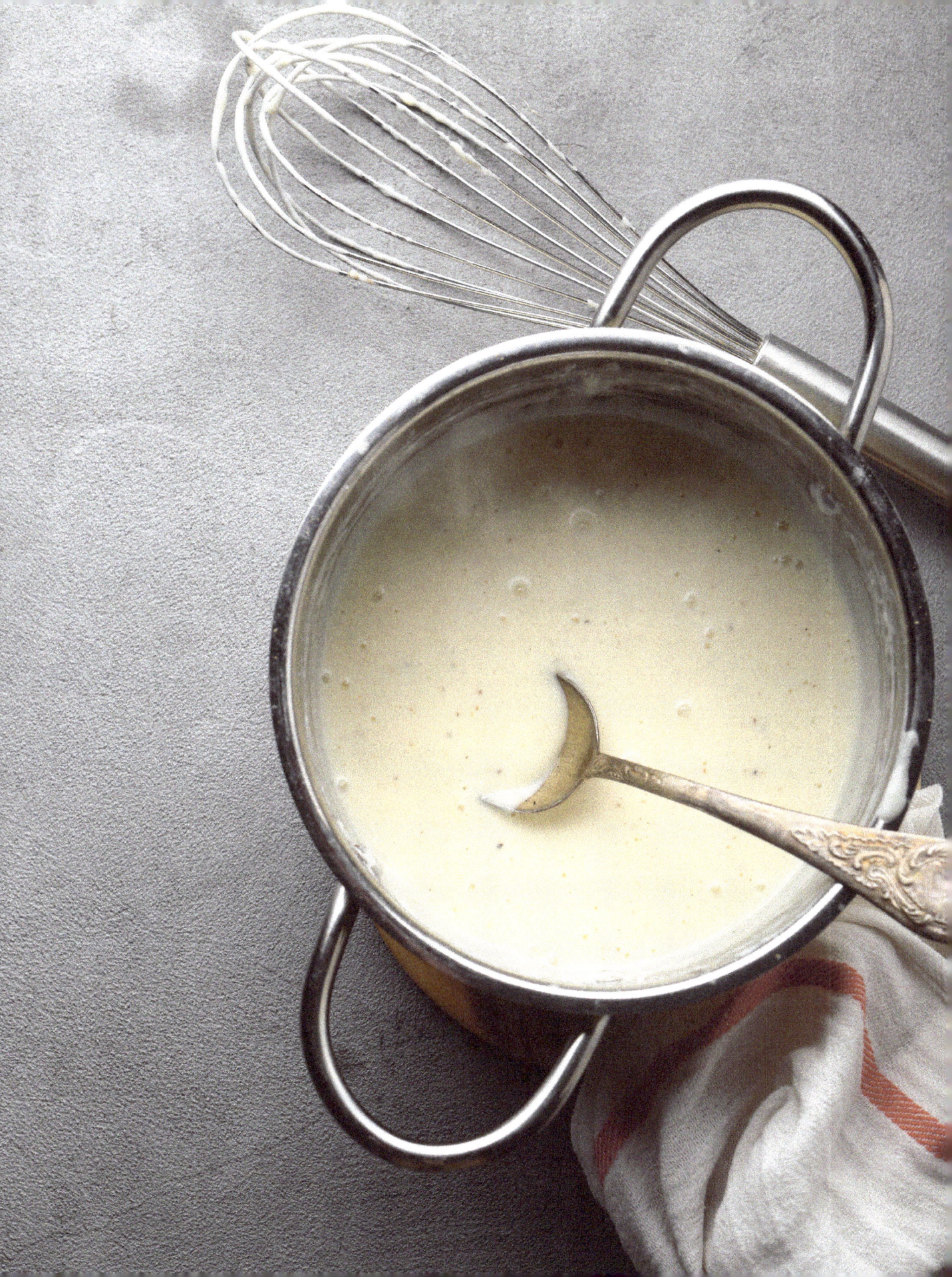

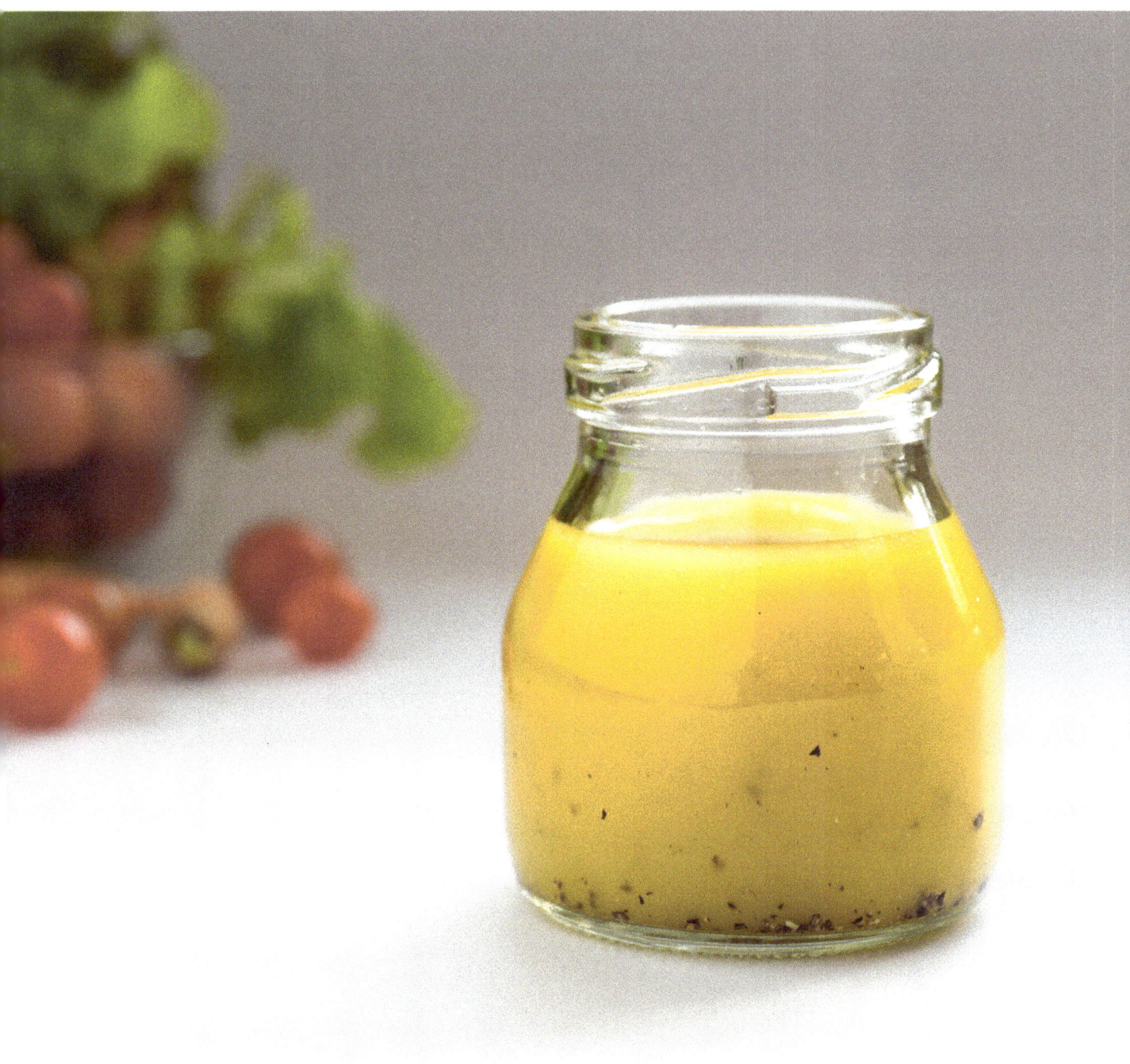

WALNUT VINAIGRETTE

**PREPARATION TIME
5 MINUTES**

INGREDIENTS:

30ml fresh lemon juice
1gm sugar
2.5gm Dijon mustard
60ml walnut oil
Himalayan sea salt/cracked pepper to taste

METHOD:

Whisk all ingredients except oil in a medium bowl. Continue to whisk while slowly adding the walnut oil in a thin stream, to thicken. Pour over desired salad.

SOUR CREAM

**PREPARATION TIME
30 MINUTES**

INGREDIENTS:

130gm raw macadamias soaked 15 minutes in hot water
80ml water
15ml lemon juice
15ml apple cider vinegar
15gm savoury yeast flakes
3gm Himalayan sea salt.

METHOD:

1. Boil water, pour over macadamias and leave for 15 minutes.
2. Drain macadamias and place in blender bowl.
3. Add all remaining ingredients.
4. Blitz all ingredients until a nice smooth consistency.
5. You may adjust seasonings to taste.

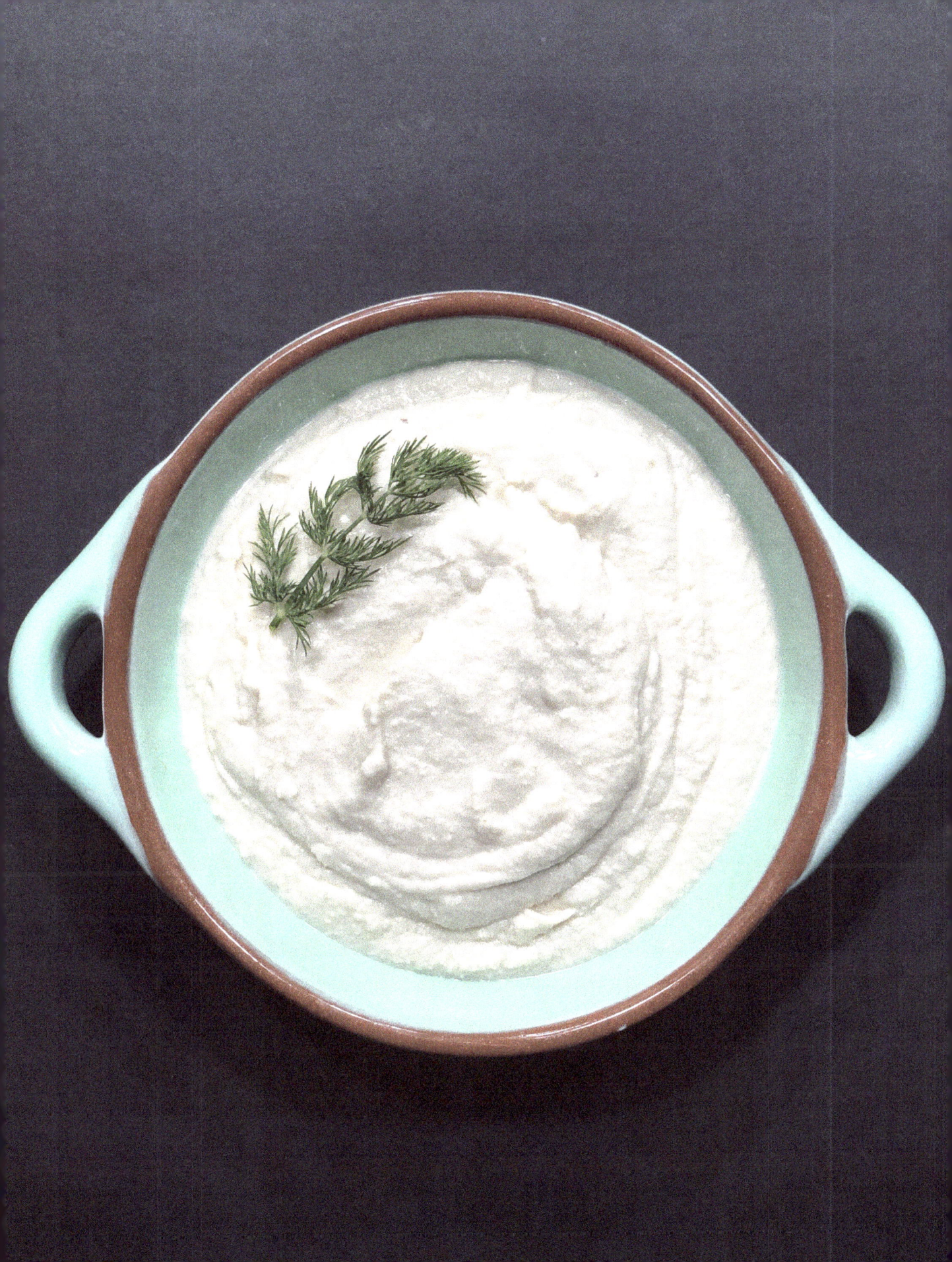

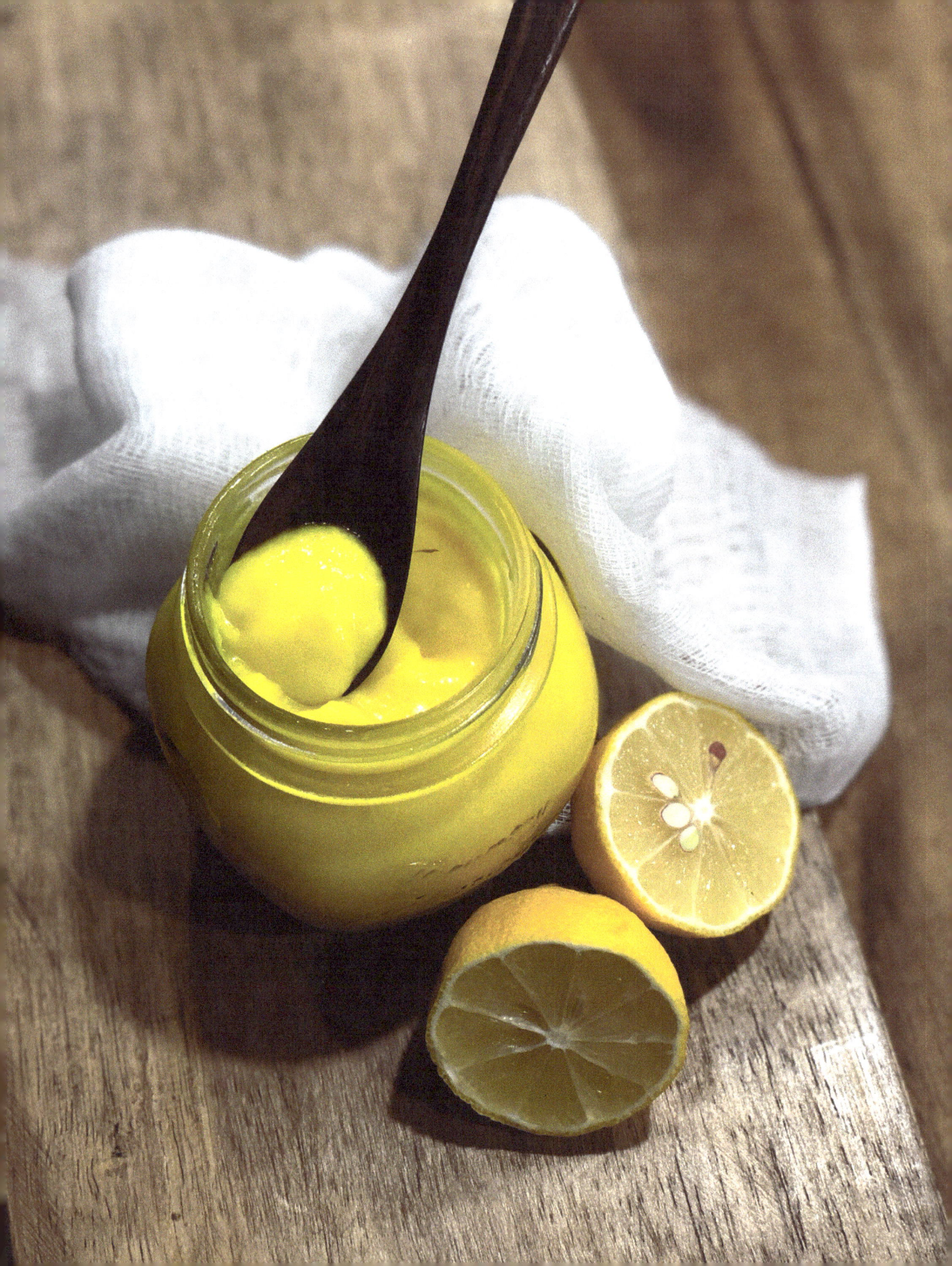

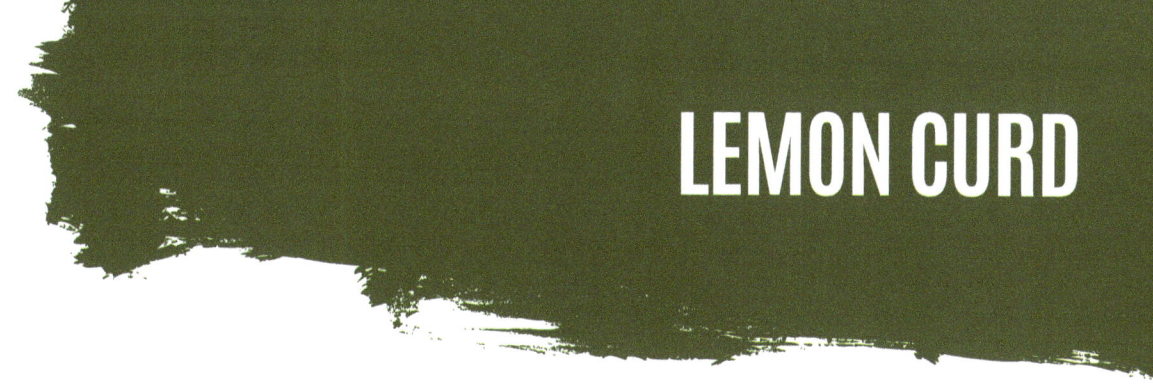

LEMON CURD

Make sure you sterilise your jar before making this little gem…

**PREPARATION TIME
15 MINUTES**

INGREDIENTS:

230gm sugar
15gm corn starch
250ml coconut milk
10gm lemon zest
125ml lemon juice
1.5gm turmeric powder

METHOD:

1. Place sugar and cornstarch in a medium saucepan and blend thoroughly.
2. Add remaining ingredients.
3. On a medium heat whisk constantly until lemon curd thickens (just to the boil).
4. Whisking constantly ensures for a nice smooth curd.
5. Remove from heat and pour into a sterilised jar.
6. Wait until it cools and keep in fridge for 1 week.
7. Curd will thicken as it cools.

MEET THE AUTHOR

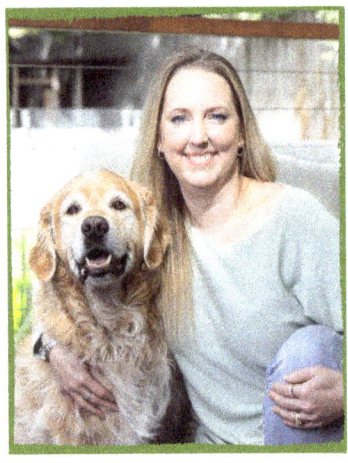

Born in Melbourne Victoria, into a wonderful loving family. I enjoyed a protected Christian upbringing that involved fun, love, laughter and togetherness. I was very much raised with the beliefs of the times, ones that weren't questioned, whether misguided or not.

Ever since I can remember I had the innate human instinct of caring and nurturing.

Some of my earliest memories are those of hearing babies cry, and I would immediately well up with them. The long arduous walks to school on a cold winter's day would involve ever so carefully picking up the worms that had been washed up on the path from the prior night's rains, so they wouldn't get stepped on or eaten by the hungry waiting birds.

From an early age I remember my grandmother taking me to visit her gorgeous aunts. At first we would visit them at their homes but before long, it was the nursing home we would frequent. Some memories of those days are vivid however some are fading. Sitting stroking my aunt's hair, while she would attempt to talk after suffering a debilitating stroke, I realised what I was supposed to do with my life.

I was going to become a nurse and change the WORLD!

True to my convictions, in 1990, my dreams came true when I excitedly enrolled to become a nurse. I remember sitting in the interview after my entrance exam with the poor result of 51% and the panel recommending I choose another career, as I would find this path difficult!

Fortunately for me as I had 'passed' the exam, they had to let me through, so I continued against their recommendations.

I LOVED IT AND I WAS GREAT AT IT

As time went on though, I became very disillusioned. Patients were numbers or categorised by their illness, there was overmedicating and not a lot of answers – it was just the way it was done.

My sister started studying naturopathy. WOW – a world was opened up to me. As passionate about health as I was, we would talk for hours about the methodology that was followed by the natural medical field. It all made sense to me. My questions were being answered and it was such a gentle, appropriate, and passive approach to illness and disease that it resonated with me greatly.

> *So after ten years, I did a backflip, left Western medicine and pursued a path in natural medicine completing my degree*
>
> *– Bachelor of Health Science – Nutritional Medicine.*

It was amazing and was filling the void I had been feeling.

After I finished my degree I spent the following two years self-studying the link between chronic illness, in particular cancer and the modern diet. After all, if we were eating what was being recommended as the standard Australian diet, then why was our race suffering more illness than ever, at a rate that is persistently escalating?

This is when it dawned on me, humans are no longer eating true to our species.

In the wild, you don't see lions, tigers, rhinos and apes full of cancer, heart disease, high cholesterol, cardiovascular disease, obesity, diverticulitis, constipation, allergies etc, etc. In our domesticated animals, because we feed them a manipulated version of their diet, do we see these diseases. They are primarily human diseases – diet and lifestyle influenced!

If this wasn't a wake-up call that, even for health reasons alone, we should be following purely a wholefoods, plant based diet, then what is? Why are we persisting with eating foods that have been proven to make us so unwell, when we can get every nutrient and phyto-nutrient from a plant-based diet? It really defies logic.

My husband of 28 years had high cholesterol and was looking down the barrel at medication. After he started on this diet, it only took six weeks before he dropped weight and lowered his cholesterol to a safe level – not one tablet taken!

With my devoted, adoring, supportive husband by my side, we now enjoy a cruelty free lifestyle, eating and sharing with our two children and extended families the amazing, tasty dishes that can be enjoyed on a wholefood, plant-based diet. Surrounded by our rescued animals, we are living true to our beliefs, ethics, morals and knowledge:

To cause no harm to the planet, the animals and especially, **OUR HEALTH...**

Hope you enjoy the recipes as much as we do,

Love Jodie

Start your day right. Every day.
With a Kuvings Vacuum Blender

Introducing,
The world's healthiest blender that locks in the nutrients by enabling you to vacuum seal the ingredients before you blend.

Why is this important?

- ✓ More nutrition
- ✓ More enzymes
- ✓ Finer & smoother texture
- ✓ Brighter, more vivid colours
- ✓ Longer lasting
- ✓ Better taste
- ✓ Less oxidation
- ✓ Less foam
- ✓ Less noise

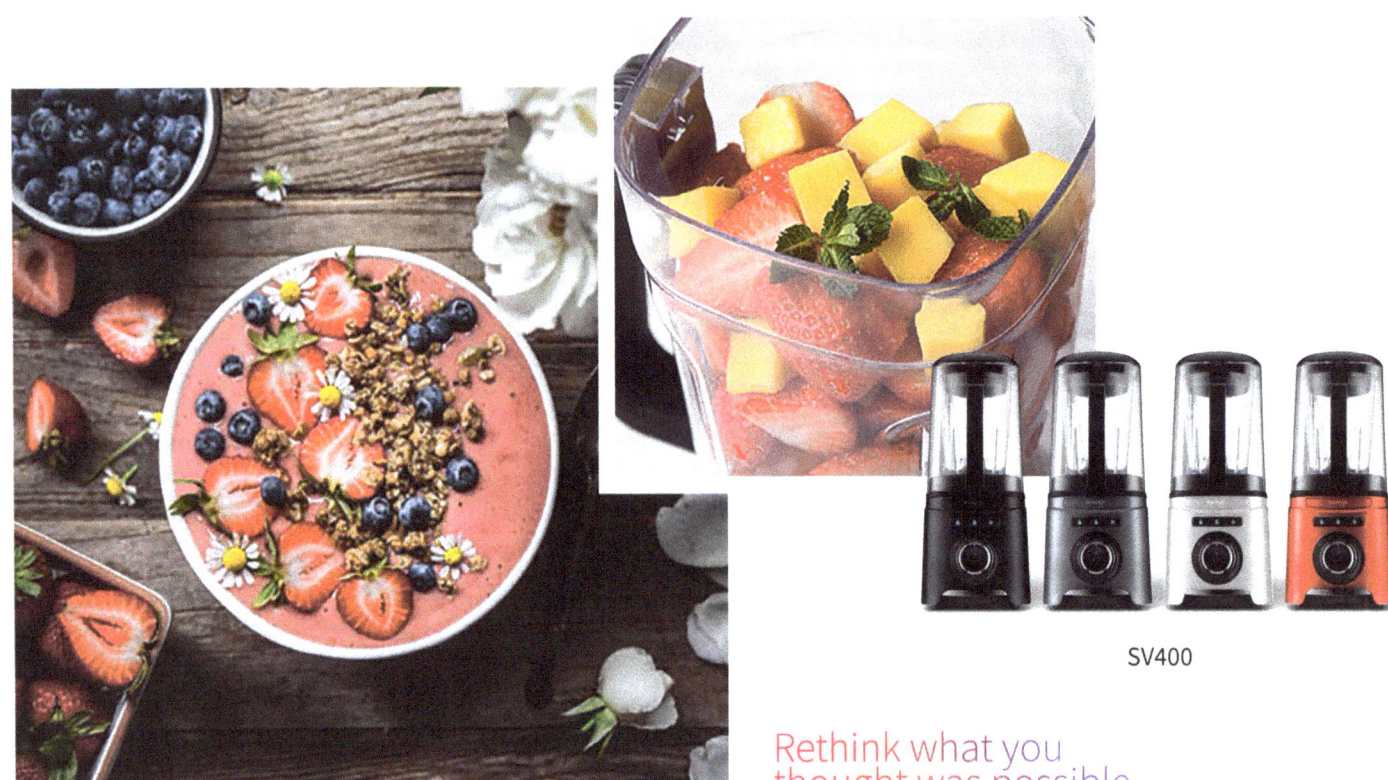

SV400

Rethink what you thought was possible

A healthy addition to any household. A Kuvings Vacuum Blender easily transforms fresh, seasonal fruits and vegetables into delicious and nutritious smoothies, dips, sauces, nut mylks and soups – simply at the touch of a button.

What's more, your daily smoothie can be made in advance when you use a Vacuum Blender. Simply vacuum seal the ingredients, store it in the fridge and it's ready for you to grab and go when you need it, without any loss of freshness or nutritional value.

Everything tastes better with a Kuvings!
www.kuvings.com.au/blenders

HOW TO TRANSITION TO A 100% PLANT BASED LIFESTYLE

Without Spending a Fortune!

Making the change can be hard, especially if you don't have someone to guide you along the way. That's why we created a specific online training program that covers everything you'll need to know when it comes to making that transition.

We've included things like:

- ✓ How to buy Healthy food quickly
- ✓ How to cook healthy meals easily that everyone will love
- ✓ How to use food as medicine
- ✓ How to eat delicious healthy food without following complicated systems
- ✓ Interviews with Leading Naturopaths
- ✓ Supplement suggestions
- ✓ Dealing with Food Allergies and food intolerances
- ✓ Juicing tips and tricks
- ✓ What superfoods to eat
- ✓ What to have in your pantry
- ✓ Organic vs Non-Organic products
- ✓ Where to shop and what to buy
- ✓ Videos, Checklists and Recipes

Plus so much more...

So to find out more go to the link below
www.Soulpodnutrition.com.au

RECOMMENDED RESOURCES

Wholefood Merchants

- 3/794 Burwood Hwy, Ferntree Gully 3156 Victoria
- 03 9752 2772
- www.wholefoodmerchants.com.au

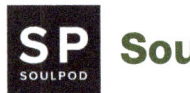 ## SoulPod Café

Croydon
- 43 The Mall, Croydon, 3136 Victoria
- 03 8488 8848

Ferntree Gully
- 3/794 Burwood Hwy, Ferntree Gully 3156 Victoria
- 03 88997891
- www.soulpodfoods.com.au

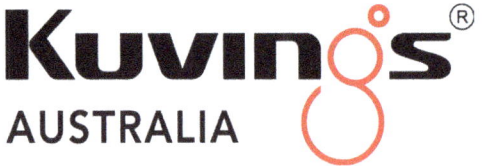

Kuvings Australia

- 1/1West Stm Croydon, 2132 NSW
- 02 9798 0586
- info@kuvings.com.au
- www.kuvings.com.au

Edgars Mission

- PO Box 270, Lancefield 3435 Victoria, Australia
- www.edgarsmission.org.au

Rabbit Runaway Orphanage

- 19 Stanley St, Olinda 3788 Victoria, Australia
- www.rabbitrunaway.org.au

RECOMMENDED RESOURCES

Healthdirect.gov.au

Badgut.org
Canadian Society of Intestinal Research

FODMAPfriendly.com

Betterhealth.vic.gov.au

RDC Clinical
rdcclinical.com.au

Monash University Gastroenterology Dept
www.monash.edu
monashfodmap.com

fodmapeveryday.com

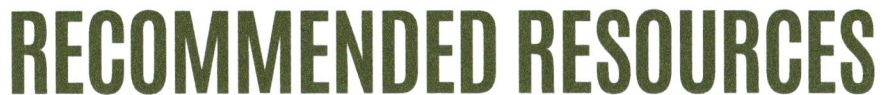

Photography thanks to Melanie Desa

Make up thanks to Rebecca Wheatley @wearitbare

www.ingramcontent.com/pod-product-compliance
Lightning Source LLC
Chambersburg PA
CBHW061209230426
43665CB00028B/2957